The V. D. Story

The V.D. Story

by

Stewart M. Brooks

1972

LITTLEFIELD, ADAMS & CO.
Totowa, New Jersey

1972 Edition

Published by LITTLEFIELD, ADAMS & CO.

By arrangement with A. S. BARNES AND CO., INC.

Printed in the United States of America

Contents

Illustrations

* These illustrations were drawn from photomicrographs in such a way that the inexperienced eye can see what the *experienced* eye sees.

Preface

Diseases passed along through the sexual act compose a very special area of medicine: they frighten us; they fascinate us. They went out of style for a decade or so during the penicillin honeymoon, but are now back again in full bloom. The purpose of this little work is to present the interested general reader with the highlights of this big subject.

Stewart M. Brooks
Waban, Mass.

Acknowledgments

Once again I wish to thank my exceptional wife, Natalie Ann Brooks, for her 24-hour assistance. Once again I wish to thank Marie Litterer for her fine art work. And once again I wish to thank all the people at A. S. Barnes & Co. for their trust, interest, and expert assistance. I am indebted to the U. S. Public Health Service's Center for Disease Control, particularly to Leslie C. Norins, M.D., Ph.D. (Chief, Venereal Disease Research Laboratory) and James B. Lucas, M.D. (Assistant Chief, Venereal Disease Branch). Also, I wish to express my appreciation to Ronald L. Bern (President, the Ronald Bern Co.), John L. Gaspar, M.D. (G. D. Searle and Co.), W. E. Rawls, M.D. (Baylor College of Medicine), Julius Schmid, Inc., and the W. B. Saunders Co.

Condoms and Conundrums

Venus was the Roman goddess of love, so not surprisingly "venereal" relates to sexual intercourse, and most especially sexual intercourse with an "infected person." Though we all tend to think of venereal disease in terms of syphilis and gonorrhea, this is by no means the complete story. The other infections in this very special category are chancroid, lymphogranuloma venereum, granuloma inguinale, trichomonas vaginitis, herpes infection, listeriosis, and last but not necessarily least to those so infected, pubic lice ("crabs").

Just exactly how many people have "V.D." is a moot question and for quite obvious reasons. Some really do not know they are sick. Some know they are sick but purposely shun the doctor. Some are far removed, geographically and otherwise, from medical facilities. Some are just plain ignorant. But first and foremost, of those *who do* show up for treatment only a pathetic few emerge as a statistic. Private physicians, those who treat 75 percent of such cases, simply do not relay the message. This, despite the fact that all states have laws requiring doctors to report each case of syphilis and gonorrhea to the proper authorities. A 1968 survey showed that these physicians report only between 10 and 20 percent of the gonorrhea cases. Thus, whereas 20,186 new cases of syphilis were diagnosed and reported to health departments in the fiscal year 1970, the Public Health Service estimated the actual figure to be between 70,000 and 80,000. And of the 573,200 reported cases of gonorrhea for fiscal 1970, the estimate is a staggering two million. According to American Medical News, outside the common cold V.D. is the No. 1 communicable disease in the United States!

The *incidence* of syphilis—the number of *new* cases occurring within a year—rose to an all time high of 106,539 in 1947 and then—thanks to penicillin—dropped to an all time low of 6,500 in 1955. Since then its *prevalence*—the *total* number of cases ("new" *and* "old")—has been on the decline, and is currently estimated to number about one-half million. But the *incidence* peaked again in 1965 (23,250 cases) and in 1970 stood at the figure cited above—20,186 cases. *Congenital* syphilis, most cases of which are somewhat paradoxically and ironically diagnosed among adults, continues to go down. In 1941 the figure stood at 17,600 (13.4 per 100,000 population) and for 1970 it was 1,903 (0.9 per 100,000). But in regard to gonorrhea the situation is a true tragedy. Whereas in 1958 there were 220,191 reported cases, giving the lowest *rate* (129.3 per 100,000 population) since 1935, the 1970 figure of 573,200 cases renders a rate of 285.2 per 100,000 population—the highest up to that year! Mincing no words the Surgeon General labels it an "epidemic," and the American Social Health Association "a pandemic."

This highly unexpected explosion has been ascribed to a concert of factors: General ignorance, relaxed sexual codes, greater mobility of population, uncooperative doctors, insufficient public health funds, and increased promiscuity among young people are all mentioned. For 1956 gonorrhea in the 15–19 age bracket stood at 45,161 cases; for 1969 the figure was 129,071 cases! And running through this epidemiologic concert is the element of complacency generated in the early days of penicillin. A shot of the magical stuff did the trick and that was that. This was the thinking of the man on the street, the doctors, the public health people, and the community at large. Thus, we dropped our guard at all levels and V.D. arose once again in full vigor and bloom.

Fortunately, complacency is now giving way to alarm, and the idea of surveillance and control is moving to front and center stage. New cases must be pinpointed at the earliest possible hour and *all contacts* searched out ("casefinding") and treated. On *all* counts and in the opinion of *all* authorities this is the basic weapon against V.D. But its success depends upon the doctors reporting *all* cases and then having enough casefinders to do the casefinding. Further, this basic theme must be embellished with a shot of real education. Certainly, the mass media help in putting across a message, but they cannot be expected to eradicate misinformation. This is a problem for the schools, and to date organized education has done a poor job of resolving the situation notwithstanding all those innovations we hear so much about. V.D. belongs in the health and science curriculums right alongside other diseases: *Clostridium tetani* causes lockjaw, *Treponema pallidum* causes syphilis, and so on.

And then, of course, there is man himself as a "preventive measure," for if he were to forswear the flesh V.D. would evaporate into nothingness. This is the ultimate. Penultimately, he can follow the dictum of the legendary "Doctor Condom" and sheath his penis in a condom. Alas, many public health people believe that the abandonment of the condom in favor of the contraceptive pill has been partly responsible for our present problems. In the words of the *Cecil-Loeb Textbook of Medicine*, a bible among the doctors, "the most effective prophylaxis against syphilis is the use of a condom during sexual intercourse and a thorough cleansing of the genitalia and adjacent areas with soap and water immediately thereafter." Thus, V.D. is a preventable unpreventable problem—and, vice versa, a conundrum if you please—and this prophylactic device deserves every consideration as a key element in solving it. And then who knows, perhaps one day the condom will carry the label—WARNING: THE SURGEON GENERAL HAS DETERMINED THAT INTERCOURSE IS DANGEROUS TO YOUR HEALTH.

The V. D. Story

SYPHILIS

1

Backgrounds

Of all the entries in the medical dictionary none compares with syphilis in sight or sound or implication: Syphilis is disease; syphilis is medicine; syphilis is history; syphilis is man. Syphilis at the very least is an institution: There is "Syphilology;" there are "Syphilogoists;" and so on. And knowing full well that a disease by any other name is just as bitter, history gives us a constellation of alternate labels: lues, plague, pox, great pox, evil pox, great mimic, Spanish disease, French disease, Italian disease, Las Bubas, and love sickness, to cite a few.

Syphilis occurs throughout the world. It is more common among the underprivileged than the privileged; more common in cities than rural areas; more common in males than females; and far more common among Blacks than Whites. No one pretends to know its true incidence and prevalence even in countries with good statistical facilities such as ours. Authorities *estimate* its prevalence in this country to be well over one-half million and its incidence to be about 80,000 new cases a year. Of the 19,130 new cases of acquired syphilis *reported* for the calendar year 1969: 6,984 were among females and 12,146 among males; 5,751 were among

Whites and 13,379 among "all other" races. For the fiscal year 1970 New Mexico led the nation with a case rate ("all stages") of 80.1 per 100,000 population. Idaho distinguished itself in the opposite direction with a case rate of 2 per 100,000 population.

Relative to mortality, the figures are obviously and frankly misleading, for deaths reported as due to other causes are frequently attributable to syphilis. Further, syphilis is often a contributory cause of death. Nonetheless, we appear to have made significant progress in this direction; that is to say, whereas the death rate was 13 per 100,000 at the turn of the century, today it is 0.3 per 100,000. And on a basis of life expectancy one study estimated that a syphilitic Negro male between 25 and 60 years receiving no appreciable treatment has his life abbreviated by about 17 percent.

Syphilis, too, is costly economically. For the year 1968 the estimated man-years of disability was 13,626 and the cost to the taxpayer for the maintenance of the syphilitic blind and insane amounted to $45 million.

Much has always been made about the origin of syphilis, a rather ambiguous concern when you stop to think about it. In the strict sense of the word, the disease would appear to have originated at the time—or close to the time—when *Treponema pallidum,* the causative microbe, arose, a "date" no one in his right mind pretends to know. In the casual and usual sense of the word, the origin of syphilis becomes a matter of history. That is, when and where was the disease first recognized as something special?

And the usual response to this query runs about as follows: Within months following the 1493 return of Columbus from his second voyage to the New World, a syphilis pandemic appeared suddenly in western Europe, which in a matter of four years engulfed the entire continent and the British Isles. Almost immediately the malady was recognized as being something really different. In 1495 Germany's Diet of Worms stamped it the *bösen blattern,* or "evil pox," and the doctors began reporting and describing the signs and symptoms. In 1530 the Veronese physician Girolamo Frascatoro published his immortal "Syphilis Sive Morbus Gallicus" ("Syphilis or French Disease"). In this medical *poem* a mythical shepherd named *Syphilus* (from the Greek *siphlos* meaning crippled or maimed) is afflicted with the "French Disease" as punishment for cursing the Gods. Frascatoro describes the disease with accuracy, underscores its venereal nature, and for posterity gave it the magical appellation Syphil*is.*

Linking the disease to Christopher Columbus was apparently the idea of one Rodrigo Ruy de Isla, a Spanish physician who in a book published in 1539 mentioned that he first recognized (years before) the signs and symptoms among the sailors of Columbus's crew. Further he attributed the affliction to the natives of Hispaniola. Those who do not go along with this so-called "columbian school" cite the syphilislike diseases of antiquity, for instance, the Biblical plague of Moab (a nation now part of Jordan). Additionally, the "pre-columbian school" puts whatever origin there is in tropical Africa.

An interesting synthesis of both schools is something like this: A primordial, nonvenereal *Treponema pallidum* of tropical Africa migrated with man to Asia, thence over the Bering Strait to America. There in the cities of Mexico and Peru it evolved into some sort of benign pathogen—a pathogen causing a *mild* venereal disease among the

Indians. Upon the arrival of the paleface, presumably Columbus and his sailors, *Treponema pallidum* suddenly went violently virulent—violently virulent enough to set off the pandemic of 1494. And so on. Historically, the pandemic of the "new disease" is well recorded; microbiologically, the switch of a pathogen from benign to virulent among new susceptibles is well recognized; and pathologically, the skeletal remains of Indians, long dead before the arrival of Columbus, disclose what is taken to be syphilitic lesions. In sum, the hypothesis is reasonable and *may* actually have been what happened.

Be that as it may, the pandemic burned itself out with the coming of the new century. Stated differently, *Treponema pallidum* became less virulent—it became the syphilis we know today. And in the context of evolution this makes much sense, because a biologically wise pathogen is not going to kill the host that feeds it. In some areas of the world, though, the moderated microbe became endemic and *nonvenereal.* "Sibbins" cropped up in Scotland in the 17th century and "spirocolon" in Greece and Russia in the 19th century. *Presently,* "bejel" occurs among the desert Arabs of the Near East, "njovera" among the Karanga people of Southern Rhodesia, "dichuchwa" among the Bantus of Bechuanaland, and "siti" in Gambia. And in our own country an epidemic of nonvenereal syphilis hit Chicago in 1949. For the most part poor economic and sociological conditions favor nonvenereal syphilis.

In the chapters to follow we shall, in some detail, talk about *Treponema pallidum,* the "disease proper," diagnosis, treatment, and prevention, in that order.

2
Treponemes

The earliest writers, the astrologers, blamed syphilis on the stars and planets and in a later age the medical men ascribed the malady to faulty humors. With the coming of the microbe the true story was soon to surface, and in the year 1905 physician Eric Hoffmann and bacteriologist Fritz Schaudinn at Berlin's renowned Reichsgesuntdheitsamt discovered *Treponema pallidum*[1] in the watery ooze of a syphilitic sore.

Treponema pallidum belongs to the spirochetes, a tribe of corkscrewlike microorganisms occupying the twilight zone between *true* bacteria (one-celled plants) and protozoa (one-celled animals).[2] Authorities are not at all certain where spirochetes belong in the microbial scheme of things and there is still much mystery regarding their

1. The biologist categorizes every living thing into a certain *Phylum*, a certain *Class* within the phylum, a certain *Order* within the class, a certain *Family* within the order, a certain *Genus* within the family, and a certain *Species* within the genus. Its scientific name is then derived from the "*Genus-species*," by convention the genus always being capitalized and both terms italicized. Thus, the spirochete of syphilis winds up in the genus "Treponema" and the species "pallidum"—hence its name *Treponema pallidum.*

2. Nonetheless, for the sake of convenience *Treponema pallidum* is officially classified as a bacterium.

life processes, even as to their mode of reproduction. The vast majority are harmless—indeed beneficial, like most microbes—and distributed widely in soil and water and the gastrointestinal tract of insects, amphibians, and mollusks. The pathogens, the harmful members, fall into three rather ill-defined groups, or genera—*Leptospira, Borrelia,* and *Treponema.* By way of important examples, the jaw breaker *Leptospira icterohaemorrhagiae* attacks the liver (Weil's disease), *Borrelia recurrentis* causes neuromuscular aches and pains and elevated temperatures (relapsing fever), and *Borrelia vincentii* (in conjunction with other organisms) is responsible for trench mouth.

Of the *treponemes* enlisting our interest, two are harmless inhabitants of the mouth, *Treponema microdentium* and *Treponema macrodentium,* and three besides *Treponema pallidum* are pathogenic: *Treponema pertenue* causes yaws (or frambesia) a vicious, ugly skin eruption of the tropics; *Treponema carateum* causes pinta, a skin condition of tropical America marked by spots encompassing all colors of the rainbow; and *Treponema cuniculi* causes rabbit syphilis, the best known instance of V.D. in animals. All of these treponemes, the good guys and the bad guys, look alike, and according to many texts *exactly* alike. Of course, looking alike by no means implies acting alike, which certainly explains in one sense at least why *Treponema pertenue* causes yaws and why *Treponema pallidum* causes syphilis.

As in all evolutionary processes there just has to be a primordial stock from which presentday pathogens arose, and the consensus is that the progenitors in the case at hand were free-living nonpathogenic forms. Stated differently, the harmless spirochetes of today are in effect

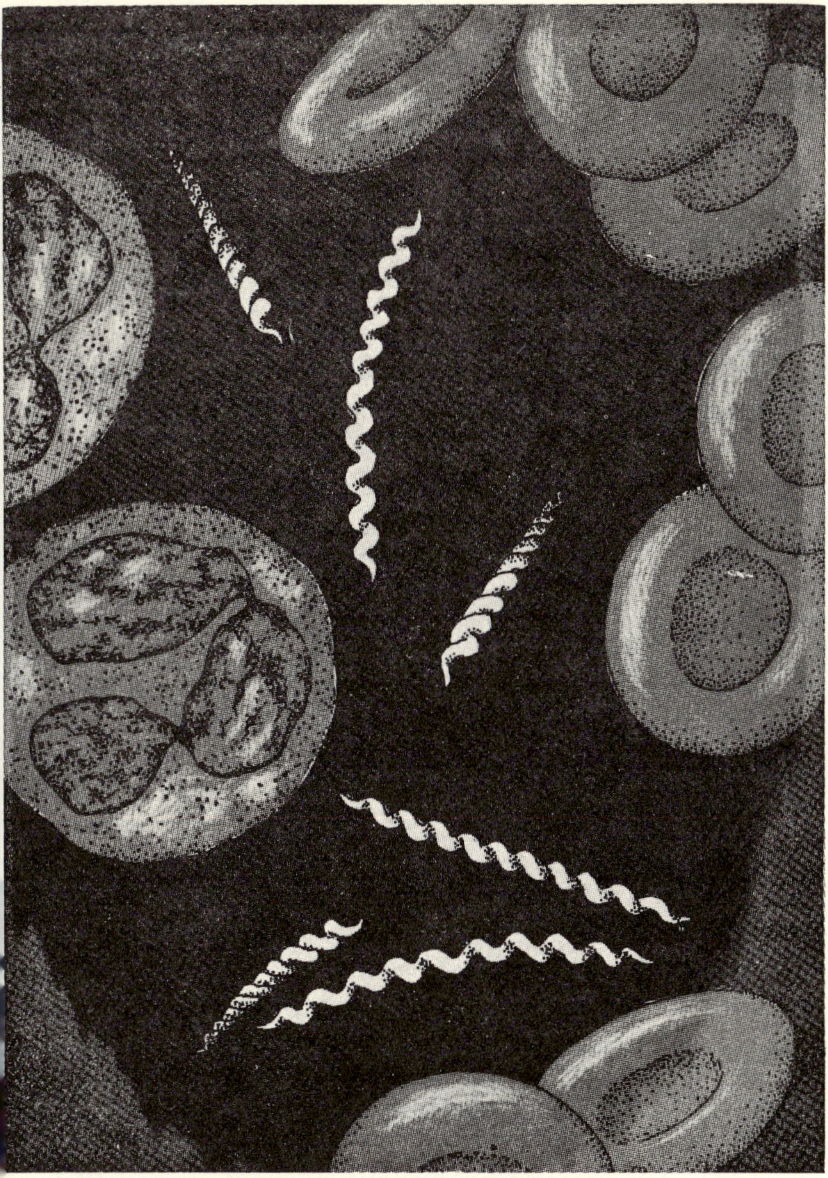

Treponema pallidum as seen through the darkfield microscope. Also very much in view are the two leukocytes (to the left) and seven red cells. (expanded 6,000x)

"living fossils," just like the horsecrab. Way back when something happened in the "survival of the fittest" department to provoke the change, most likely something happened relative to the environment. For instance, maybe some innocuous spirochete migrated from its birthplace in the tropics to the inhospitable climes of North America and once there "went venereal" in order to stay alive—that is to say, it became *Treponema pallidum.*

Treponema pallidum has a flexible cylindrical body twisted into a dozen or so regular, sharp spirals. The ends are pointed. It is very long as microbes go, about twice as long as the diameter of a red blood cell, but unbelievably thin. More precisely, a typical treponeme of the species runs about 16 microns in length and 0.3 micron in width.[3] As a matter of fact, *Treponema pallidum* is so skinny that the usual staining methods used to visualize microorganisms are of no avail. And as the student of high school biology well knows, unstained microorganisms are commonly impossible to see under the microscope. But the Austrian-American biologist Karl Landsteiner solved the staining problem (in 1909) in the most ingenious way. Instead of viewing the treponemes in light coming up directly through the specimen, he blocked out these central rays and employed strong *lateral* illumination. This makes the subject appear bright against a *dark* background, just as dust particles in the air become visible when a ray of sunlight passes through a darkened room.

Darkfield microscopy, as Landsteiner's technique became known, affords the added feature of allowing the subject to be viewed alive and moving—stains kill!—a

3. One micron, a microscopic unit of length, equals 1/25,400 inch.

tremendous advantage in the instance of *Treponema pallidum.* This notorious microbe may indeed look like its relatives, but it certainly gets about in a most characteristic fashion. Its movements are slight and slow and stately and almost always unhurried. The driving force, the motor, is a "turning of the screw" and this is exactly the way these treponemes appear in the darkfield—silvery corkscrews majestically turning and twirling their way along. Too, there may be bending and buckling and accordion-like compression and expansion of their coils and loops. Occasionally, there is a rapid quivering motion of a wire spring. All in all it is one of the best shows microscopy has to offer.

Microbiologists have succeeded in culturing artificially (outside human or animal hosts) just about every kind of microorganism except *Treponema pallidum.* Several researchers using sophisticated tissue cultures have claimed otherwise, but the general feeling has been that most or all reported culturings involve treponemal impostors—lookalikes which *do not* cause syphilis. On the authority of the U. S. Public Health Service's Venereal Disease Research Laboratory, there have as of this date been no successful culturings of *Treponema pallidum.*

Coming to the point, to our concern here, *Treponema pallidum* grows well in two places—in the tissues of man and in the testicles of the experimental rabbit. In these hospitable environments it reproduces by splitting in half every 30 hours or so. Usually it splits transversely but upon occasion perhaps longitudinally.

Heat, sunlight, dehydration, oxygen, soap, distilled water, and the usual antiseptics destroy *Treponema pallidum* in minutes and generally in seconds; "moderate" temperatures destroy it in a matter of hours. A temperature of 102°F. kills *Treponema pallidum* in five hours and 104°F. in three hours! Fragility, then, is a physiologic feature of very special note and completely explains the difficulty in culturing the organism artificially. Above all it completely explains why close contact–sexual intercourse, kissing a syphilitic sore–is a must in the spread of syphilis!

3
Stages

Syphilis is a tremendously complicated pathologic affair; most other infections are what you might call simple or straightforward in comparison. For good reason history dubs it the "great imitator," and none other than Sir William Osler, a later day Hippocrates, counseled, "Know syphilis and you will know medicine." It has taken centuries to break the mysterious ice and even today the cellular and molecular details are vexatiously baffling, albeit fascinatingly so.

The first major book on the disease was penned in 1498 by a Spanish poet-physician named Francisco Lopez de Villalobos. This man recognized the venereal mode of transmission and described with much clarity the skin eruptions and later complications. In 1514 another Spaniard, Juan de Vigo, delineated certain stages of syphilis in his "Le Mal François," and in the year 1530 Frascatoro came along with his immortal "Syphilis Sive Morbus Gallicus." Niccolo Massa, an Italian physician, underscored certain neurological ramifications of the affliction in 1532, and in 1579 William Clowes became the first investigator to broach the subject in the English language. In France, Armand Trousseau took note of the disease in pregnancy (1846) and a few years later, in 1854, Pierre Diday published a nearly complete account of what medicine was to call congenital or prenatal syphilis. But the best remembered student of the latter area of the disease was the English surgeon Sir Jonathan Hutchinson (1828–1913). His studies on the stigmata of late congenital syphilis are classic and such expressions as "Hutchinson's teeth" and "Hutchinson's triad" continue to grace the pages of pathology. The French dermatologist Jean Alfred Fournier (1832–1914) was the first investigator to stress the fact that syphilis is a smoldering infection, a concept embraced by the word *latency*. Fournier clarified scores of misconceptions and proved for the first time that general paralysis of the insane arose from antecedent syphilis.

All of this sounds more or less like steady progress, climbing up the ladder of knowledge so to speak. But evolution and history do not really operate this way and the classic example in the instance of syphilis concerns the "contribution" of England's John Hunter, a medical giant of the 18th century. Although basically an anatomist and surgeon, Hunter—like most doctors of the time—was much interested in venereal disease and set out to investigate the relationship between "the Spanish disease" and gonorrhea. And so in the year 1767 he inoculated himself with pus from a "gonorrhea patient" and lo and behold the great surgeon developed not only gonorrhea but syphilis as well, the latter ultimately causing his death in 1793. In other words—and unbeknown to Hunter, of course—this most historic pus was coincidentally swarming with the germs of *both* diseases. And thus at a time when many doctors were beginning to seriously question the "duality concept" (that gonorrhea was the initial sign of syphilis) Sir John came along with solid and influential support of the idea. His "Treatise on Venereal Diseases" (1787), embroidering and embellishing his findings, became the bible of the day and managed quite well in setting back the clock a good half century. Benjamin Bell's "Treatise on Gonorrhea Virulenta and Lues Venera" (1793) clearly proclaimed the distinctness of the two conditions (based upon experimentation on himself and his medical students), but not until the French physician Philippe Ricord published his researches in 1838 was the matter essentially put to rest. Ricord's work entailed an unbelievable 2,500 inoculations, each of which in no uncertain terms brought to light the fallacy of duality. Additionally, this perspicacious pursuing of the truth carefully characterized the stages of syphilis and provided the terms still used in the classification of the disease—primary, secondary, tertiary. Indeed, we shall now consider these stages in some detail—and from start to finish.

Treponema pallidum is, as we know, a most fragile and sensitive microbe. It needs living tissue and just the right amount of light and warmth and moisture. And even then its chances for survival are not good in unfamiliar surroundings. Put bluntly, man must go out of his way to infect himself in the instance of *acquired* syphilis. The congenital variety is a different story, and one we shall talk about in some detail once we have explored the venereal version.

Sexual intercourse is figuratively and literally a juicy affair and provides made-to-order physical and chemical conditions. The treponemes find a nice place to swim about and the frenzied, forceful movement of the penis against the vaginal walls quite apparently is sufficient to force them through the skin and mucous membranes. And here, incidentally, we find considerable equivocation among the textbooks. Some say that treponemes cannot penetrate *intact* skin and mucous membranes (mucosa), others that treponemes cannot penetrate intact skin but can penetrate mucous membranes, and still others that treponemes can penetrate both. The most reasonable view seems to be this: Treponemes cannot pass through truly intact skin, but probably do, under the right conditions, pass through intact mucosa. Comparing skin to mucosa is much like comparing cement to tissue paper. But water seeps through cracked cement, and biologic secretions charged with treponemes easily seep through skin lesions—the *micro*scopic as well as the *macro*scopic. And a lesion of the mucosa, of course, affords a pathologic avenue par excellence. In sum, if one partner in the sex act possesses a syphilitic sore, say on the penis or vaginal wall, and the other possesses a break in the skin or mucosa, an enterprising treponeme or two—and it takes only one—can gain entrance and proceed to cause trouble.

The genitals are not uniquely susceptible to infection, however, and any form of intimate body contact "suffices" if it involves the transfer of liquid infectious material. Kissing and abnormal sex practices are recognized modes of transfer and initial syphilitic lesions upon occasion involve the lips, tongue, tonsils, eyelids, breasts, and fingers. *Indirect* transfer is possible and sometimes probable, particularly among doctors, nurses, and laboratory people who handle infectious material and contaminated instruments. Infection, too, has been transmitted by blood transfusions. But otherwise the indirect situation is quite unlikely and the patient who blames the toilet seat begs the proverbial pun—It's a damn poor place to have intercourse!

We wish now to turn our microscopic spotlight on the handful of treponemal invaders. Right away they start to "multiply by division" at the site of inoculation, and before long are steadily making their way into the lymph vessels and bloodstream, a total spirochetemia[1] prevailing within a matter of 24 hours. For days and weeks and months and years these microbial corkscrews ply this scarlet humor and eventually travel to the "ends of the body" where they screw their way through the capillaries and set up new localizations (foci) of infection. Conceivably such very tiny creatures could do no harm, but the sad truth is they do. Above all and regardless of the tissue in question the response (to the invader) is fundamentally the same throughout the body—to wit, inflammation of the linings of the arteries followed by collapse and closure of the smaller branches (a condition known to pathology as obliterative endarteritis). Too, there is a great deal of tissue hypersensitivity and abundant fibrosis (overdevelopment of fibrous tissue). These forces in concert with probably countless other morbid elements *eventually* plunge the affected areas into structural and functional darkness.

And so "at 24 hours" the invader has invaded and mischief is afoot, but the victim does not feel a thing. And he is not going to feel—or *see*—anything throughout the so-called primary *incubation* period, a period running anywhere from a few days to a few months. The average is about three weeks.

Now the chancre appears—the hallmark of *primary*

1. Presence of spirochetes in the blood.

syphilis—at the site of inoculation ("portal of entry") and the reason why it occurs here and not elsewhere (at other foci) relates to seniority, the treponemes at this location having had the longest time to cause trouble. The usual sites of development are the penis and scrotum in the male, and the vulva, vagina, and cervix in the female, but extragenital lesions, as indicated earlier, are not uncommon. As a matter of fact, among homosexuals the anal chancre is on the upswing. Interestingly, *many* patients are unable to give a history of this signal primary lesion and some clinicians go so far as to say that the chancre does indeed fail to develop in about a quarter of all cases of the disease. The consensus, however, seems to be that the chancre develops in practically all cases of acquired syphilis, but is often overlooked because of its banal character or location. The cervical chancre is a classic example, the patient neither seeing it nor feeling it.

Typically, chancres are single rather than multiple. The lesion is round with a firm base and raised border and varies in size from a pinhead to the tip of the thumb, the average diameter being slightly less than half an inch. The surface appears eroded rather than ulcerated and gentle pressure calls forth a watery discharge rather than pus. Typically, too, the genital lesion *does not* pain, itch, or burn. Extragenital chancres tend to be larger and quite painful. Commonly, the chancre of syphilis is referred to as a "hard" or "huntarian" chancre (after John Hunter) to distinguish it from the so-called "soft" chancre (chancroid), a very special venereal disease caused by a very special germ (and to be discussed later on).

Another characteristic feature of primary syphilis is the development of buboes, or swollen regional lymph nodes, an event occasioned by the lymphatic drainage system; that is, treponemes in the chancre area enter the lymph vessels leading to these nodes and there set off an inflammatory response, just as they did at the portal of entry. The textbook picture in the instance of the genital chancre is the development of buboes in *both* groins (bilateral lymphadenitis).[2] Buboes and chancres are alive with treponemes!

Aside from the chancre and lymphadenitis, the patient is entirely well. Occasionally there is a slight temperature and headache (the latter indicating an invasion of the central nervous system), but *at this time* is of little or no consequence. In a month or so the chancre heals—with or *without* treatment—leaving a pale scar. Lymphadenitis, *if* it occurs, may resolve itself or it may persist and become more prominent in the secondary stage. But probably the most important point to keep in mind is that the victim of syphilis may very well pass through the primary stage without knowing it, and such is often the case when the chancre is trivial or hidden away out of sight.

The passing of the chancre heralds the end of the primary stage and the beginning of the secondary incubation period, during which time the treponemes are swimming about in increasing numbers and setting up all sorts of pathologic campsites throughout the body. This goes on for weeks or months (the average time is about six weeks) until one day the patient arrives at the *secondary* stage, the emblems of which are a generalized skin eruption (usually including the palms and soles) and "mucous patches." The rash is highly varied and may simulate almost any skin lesion—measles for instance—

2. Inflammation of lymph glands (nodes).

and there is no itching. In the typical case (if there is such a thing), the mucous patches appear a couple of weeks or so following the appearance of the rash. These are circular, multiple areas of erosion on the mucous membranes of the mouth, throat, genitalia, and rectum. About a half inch in size, they are at first red and flat and then rather suddenly turn gray and ulcerate. Mucous patches teem with treponemes and are the most infectious lesion of syphilis, not excepting the chancre. Other secondary features *usually* present are lymphadenitis (often a carryover from the primary stage) and raised, table-topped or mushroomlike papules about the genitalia or rectum called condyloma lata. On close inspection these structures appear whitish and soggy and frequently coalesce into plaquelike forms. Like the mucous patches they make their appearance following the skin eruption and once present, persist for months.

Much less common, but nonetheless of special note in putting the diagnostic finger on the secondary stage, are diffuse, patchy, falling out of hair (alopecia areata), inflammation of the iris (syphilitic iritis), pain in the shin bone (periostitis), and a slight involvement of the brain and spinal cord. Constitutional symptoms are almost always mild and almost always overlooked, especially in men. That is to say, the low grade fever, general aches and pains, and/or sickish feeling is commonly passed off for just about anything save the disease of syphilis.

The signs and symptoms of the secondary stage last anywhere from six weeks to six months and then disappear—with or *without* treatment. Recurrences are possible but nowadays uncommon because one or two doses of penicillin literally annihilate the treponemes. Before penicillin relapsing lesions invariably meant therapeutic failure; today relapsing lesions invariably mean *reinfection.* Stated another way, in order to get syphilis a second time the victim must be *completely cured the first time,* and the reason why this is true amounts to the sum and substance of a real understanding of the disease. More to the point, it explains the events which follow the secondary stage.

Long, long ago it was discovered that a person infected with syphilis rarely contracted the disease again, especially if the infection were of long standing. That is to say, subsequent encounters with *Treponema pallidum* typically do not lead to a replay of the stage or stages already passed through. In short, an infected individual is immune to *foreign* treponemes and to a pronounced degree he is immune to his own treponemes, so immune in fact that *two-thirds* of the patients emerging from the secondary stage live out their lives clinically free of signs and symptoms—and with or *without* treatment! The other third or so go on to *tertiary,* or late, syphilis and only about 15 percent of these people develop signs and symptoms from their tissue involvements. To fully appreciate all this let us briefly explore the subject of resistance.

Whenever a foreign agent (called an antigen) enters the body certain cells in the lymph nodes and other areas respond by producing and releasing to the blood *neutralizing* chemical factors called antibodies. Just how this is done is a moot question and for our purpose let us simply say that antigen X stimulates the cells to produce antibody Y, and so on. In some infections the neutralizing or inhibiting antibody is phenomenally and fantastically effective. The measles virus, for example, stimulates such a high concentration of effective antibody that

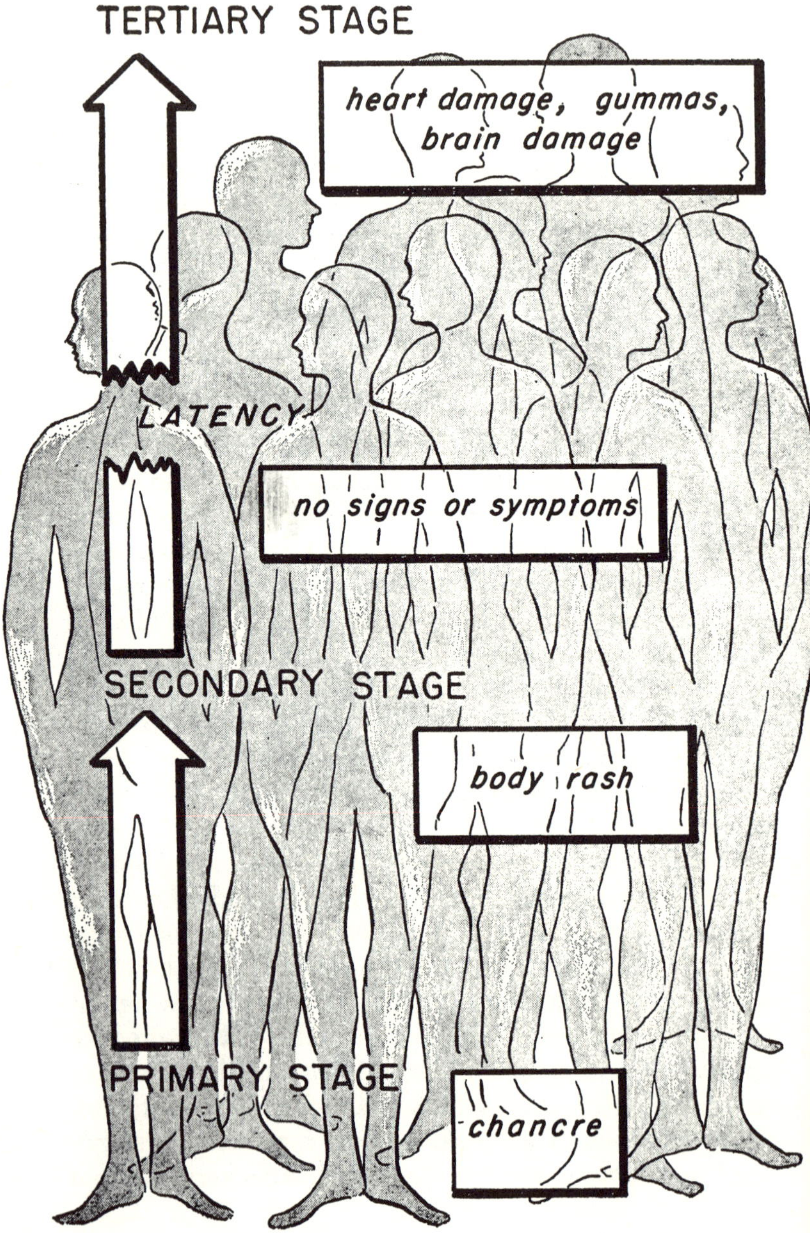

The stages of syphilis.

an attack of the disease engenders a life-long immunity. Unfortunately, the immunity encountered in syphilis is neither this simple nor dramatic. *Treponema pallidum* does indeed stimulate the production of antibodies but a great deal of research points to several other immune mechanisms. Actually, resistance to syphilis seems to depend chiefly upon some obscure cellular changes which render the tissues unfavorable for the organism. Thus, "domestic treponemes" call into play a concert of defense forces against "foreign treponemes"—thereby preventing *reinfection*—and such a state of affairs continues to prevail just as long as these domestic treponemes are about to keep said forces on their toes. Alas, once the patient is cured—that is, once all treponemes are eradicated—he is no more immune to the disease than he was the first time!

Above all, the defense mechanisms operating against foreign treponemes are, as already indicated, good enough against domestic treponemes to prevent the development of tertiary, or late, syphilis in two-thirds of those afflicted. Clearly, there is a deadly struggle going on between host and parasite, a struggle destined to last a year, a decade—or a lifetime! No one can predict how long it will last or what the outcome will be, because it all depends on the unforeseen natural forces sequestered within the substance of the body and the treponeme itself. The victim is quite unaware of these smoldering microscopic engagements and is, as the doctors so laconically say, "asymptomatic." In the language of syphilology he is passing through the twilight of *latency*, the period or interval between the secondary and tertiary stages. Among those who *do not* develop the tertiary features (and this is the majority) the latent period turns out to be "something" with a beginning but apparently no "practical" end. The textbooks are not too clear on this point. But for the sake of argument it does seem reasonable to assume in such cases that the latent period for most intents and purposes is life-long.

Lest the reader not see the forest because of the many trees and in way of review of the situation up to this point: Intimate contact introduces treponemes through a break in the skin or mucosa, thus setting up a base camp from which they (the treponemes) and their progeny set out to invade the body at large via the lymph vessels and bloodstream. On good authority a full blown spirochetemia prevails at the end of 24 hours. Treponemal activity becomes intense—"multiplication by division," screwing in and out of the capillaries, cellular destruction, and so on—and in about three weeks there is an outbreak at the site of inoculation in the form of the hard chancre. The patient typically feels fine and by the end of six weeks or so the chancre has disappeared. The patient is now without signs and symptoms of any kind for about six weeks or so, at which time enough treponemal malfeasance has accrued to bring up the curtain on the second stage—skin rash, mucous patches, and so on. These lesions usually persist for an average of twelve weeks or thereabouts and with their disappearance the patient enters the latent period, a period lasting anywhere from a year to a lifetime. *It all depends on the outcome of the continuing battle between the treponemes and the forces of immunity.* Some one-third of afflicted individuals pass into the tertiary, or late, stage of the disease. . . . This is the picture of the evolution and natural history of syphilis in the *absence* of treatment. What happens in the wake of a shot of penicillin is a critical topic of a future chapter.

With the aforesaid keenly in mind, let us now turn to the reverberations and repercussions of tertiary syphilis, the last link in the long journey from the chancre to the disease's morbid conclusions. Statistically, about one-quarter of untreated patients entering this stage can be expected to die primarily as a result of treponemal activity; cardiovascular complications account for the great bulk (a good 80 percent) of the deaths. And by far and away the cardinal lesion is an inflammatory scarring and weakening of the aorta, the great vessel taking blood away from the heart's left ventricle. Commonly, the valve guarding the opening between these two structures is damaged, causing a leaking back (regurgitation) of blood. The result is compensatory overwork, enlargement, and heart failure. Other ominous possibilities include an outpouching (aneurysm) of the aortic arch (rupture of which causes a fatal hemorrhage) and a direct treponemal attack against the heart muscle proper.

The majority of the remaining deaths in tertiary syphilis relate to the central nervous system (neurosyphilis), the basic forms of which are characterized as meningeal, meningovascular, tabetic, and paretic. According to the very latest thinking, the groundwork for these pathetic involvements is quite well established in the *early* weeks of the disease, this idea fitting in very nicely with the occasional case of the primary disease marked by *clinical* neurosyphilitic overtones. Stated another way, neurosyphilis starts early or it does not start at all. But irrespective of the particular kind of pathology, nervous system dysfunction *always* commences with an attack on the meninges (the membranous wrappings about the brain and spinal cord), the expression *meningeal* neurosyphilis being specially reserved for those cases of the disease where the treponemes have not gone beyond said wrappings. The signs and symptoms are headache, stiff neck, and sometimes paralysis of facial muscles. *Meningovascular* neurosyphilis involves both the meninges and the blood vessels (of the nervous system) and consequently portends the likelihood of varying degrees of damage to the spinal cord and brain tissue.

Tabetic neurosyphilis arises from a treponemal attack on the substance of the spinal cord, the sequelae encompassing a progressive wasting away of the body together with crises of intense pain, incoordination, peculiar sensations, loss of reflexes, and sudden, violent functional disturbances of the various organs. Urinary retention and concomitant urinary tract infections are common, and about one out of ten tabetics develop optic nerve degeneration leading to blindness. The term tabetic, incidentally, comes from the Latin *tabes,* meaning "wasting away," and *tabes dorsalis*—a somewhat older expression for tabetic neurosyphilis—refers to the fact that the damage is confined to the back, or *dorsal,* part of the spinal cord. Further, because of the muscular incoordination (ataxia) there are ambulatory difficulties, accounting for the much older expression *locomotor ataxia.* Of much diagnostic importance in this tragic state of affairs, whatever we call it, are characteristic deformities of the joints ("Charcot joints") and constricted irregular pupils which do not respond to light. The latter phenomenon—known to medicine as the "Argyll Robertson pupil"—is a hallmark of neurosyphilis in general and tabetic neurosyphilis in particular.

Paretic neurosyphilis, or general paresis, arises from a treponemal invasion of the brain, and in interesting contrast to other tertiary features this very special organ discloses treponemes in large numbers. Upon autopsy the

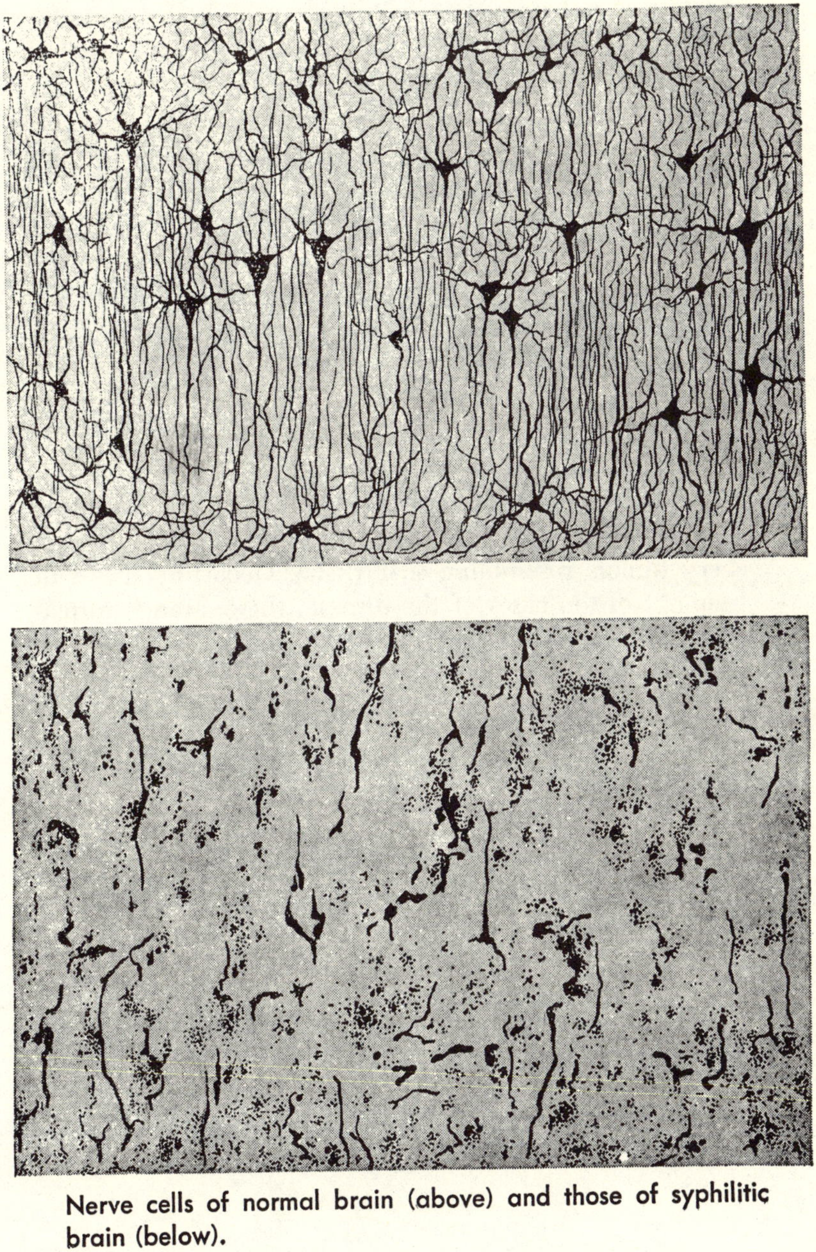

Nerve cells of normal brain (above) and those of syphilitic brain (below).

brain is noted to have shrunk away from its bony casing and the lining of the ventricles (the small cavities within the brain) are highly granulated rather than clear and smooth. Microscopically there is considerable dishevelment of the cerebral cortex (the outer portion of the cerebrum) and widespread loss of nerve cells, a tissue picture one standard textbook of pathology dubs as "windswept." The clinical reflections of this very overt injury are gradual and progressive, beginning with subtle changes in the intellect, memory, mood, behavior, and such, and ending in very extraordinary dementing psychoses. The terminal individual is quivering and trembling and insane. He is the quintessence of all that the disease syphilis has to offer.

Aside from—but certainly in addition to—the gruesome details related above, is the matter of *gummas,* soft rubbery tumors resembling scar tissue. Occurring in about one out of ten cases of the disease, these strange formations are considered by most authorities to be an allergic response to the invader. The location, number, and effects of these lesions are extremely varied and along with the cardiovascular and nervous ramifications make syphilis the "great imitator" that it is. In many areas, such as the liver and spleen, gummas cause little trouble but in the event of bone involvement fractures and joint destruction are not uncommon.

And let us turn now to the congenital, or prenatal, version of the great imitator.

The fetus "acquires" syphilis as a consequence of the migration of treponemes across the so-called "placental barrier," where maternal blood and fetal blood are only a capillary away, so to speak. Such an invasion generally occurs after the fifth month of pregnancy. In early syphilis, pregnancy practically always results in miscarriage, stillbirth, and diseased babies. And quite to the contrary, women who become pregnant many years after infection often give birth to normal babies. Or, to put it another way, the likelihood of the fetus being infected decreases with the duration of the mother's infection.

"Congenital babies" are not likely to show evidence of disease until a good three or four weeks of age, at which time some sort of skin eruption can almost always be depended upon to appear. The most typical lesion is what the physician calls a maculopapular rash; that is, a combination of discolored flat (maculo-) and raised (-papular) spots. These are characteristically patterned about the face and mouth, palms, soles, and anogenital region; the papular spots are often grouped together and often infected. Other eruptive manifestations are mucous patches in the mouth and condylomatous lesions (very similar to those of acquired syphilis) about the anus and genitals. And the appearance on the hands and soles of bullae—large blisters—is specifically distinctive. Finally, all moist lesions, regardless of their location, are potentially infectious.

Other marks of distinction in the early days of the disease are cracking of the lips, enlarged spleen, snuffles, and peculiar cry. The cracking becomes embellished by well defined fissures radiating in a sunburst manner about the mouth, often extending a half inch or so from the lips. In the wake of the healing process these fissures leave telltale scars called rhagades (from the Greek *rhagas*, meaning rent). The spleen often undergoes enormous enlargement, producing the well recognized "potbelly." The snuffles, or catarrhal nasal discharge, is sometimes bloody, and the inaudible or "cracked-pot" cry is actually a pronounced laryngitis. And in regard to overall appearance, the syphilitic infant is puny and withered and shriveled with the face of a little old man.

Whether or not the infected infant develops these early signs and symptoms, he does indeed develop the late or "juvenile lesions" at an average age of 10 years or so. The classic feature here is Hutchinson's *triad*—inflammation of the cornea of the eye (often resulting in blindness), deafness (due to auditory nerve damage), and notching of the upper central incisors (Hutchinson's teeth). Additionally, there are considerable and widespread skeletal changes, resulting in such characteristic developments as a sunken bridge of the nose ("saddle nose"), forward curve of the tibial bones ("saber shins"), enlarged forehead, and painless symmetrical enlargement of the joints, particularly of the knees ("Clutton's joints"). Cardiovascular lesions are rare, but neurosyphilis is not uncommon and may appear in the same forms as noted in the adult. Juvenile paresis—insanity and paralysis in the child—is the star attraction in *Treponema pallidum's* chamber of horrors.

4
Tests

To establish whether a chancre is really a chancre or a mucous patch is really a mucous patch, all one need do is examine a drop of exudate for the presence of treponemes. The routine procedure here is darkfield microscopy, but there is every reason to believe that the very recent Fluorescent Antibody Darkfield (FADF) test or some related technique will gain popularity either as a supplement or substitute. Nonmotile or insufficient numbers of treponemes and artifacts make interpretation of some darkfield examinations difficult. Also, darkfield preparations are seldom attempted on oral lesions due to indigenous treponemes which are difficult to differentiate from *Treponema pallidum,* even by experienced personnel. Hence, the interest in FADF. The gist of the test is as follows: Syphilitic antibody combined and "tagged" with the fluorescent dye fluorescein is added to a smear of the exudate (on a glass slide) and then rinsed gently in water to remove the excess. If treponemes are indeed present they will "absorb" the antibody and glow beautifully when viewed through the ultraviolet microscope. This does not happen with any other organism because syphilitic antibody combines only with *Treponema pallidum.*

Unhappily, the diagnosis of syphilis is seldom this straightforward, for well over three-quarters of the syphilitic patients seen by the doctor are in latency. In this period, as we have learned, there is nothing in the way of a clinical picture and, in addition, the treponemes are few and far between and just about impossible to locate and demonstrate. This situation obtains in other bacterial infections, too, but usually the laboratory people can culture a pathogen to the point of "having plenty to work with." For example, even though a specimen may contain only one or two streptococci the appropriate culture medium can expand this figure into the millions in a matter of hours. To date no one has developed such a culture medium for the propagation of *Treponema pallidum.*

And so it boils down to this: The diagnosis of syphilis centers upon what medicine calls serology, or the study of antigen-antibody reactions *in vitro* (that is, "in the test tube"). More particularly, it means taking the patient's blood serum (the clear liquid which separates from the cells in the clotting process) and searching for telltale antibodies. And this is a story in itself, a story dating back to the year 1898.

In that year the Belgian bacteriologist Jules Bordet, discovered a certain protein substance in blood serum called complement, an agent which apparently bonds itself to any and all antigen–antibody complexes.[1]

Moreover, in some antigen–antibody reactions Bordet

1. As used here a complex refers to the chemical union between an antigen and antibody formed in a so-called antigen–antibody reaction.

found that complement[2] was an essential element! To cite the classic experiment, when sheep red cells (antigen) are injected into the bloodstream of the rabbit, the latter's immunity system responds by producing an antibody called hemolysin. In the *absence* of complement, hemolysin does not affect red cells; in the *presence* of complement, hemolysin destroys red cells. Thus, when rabbit serum containing anti-sheep hemolysin—and complement—is added to a watery suspension of sheep red cells the mixture immediately turns a clear pinkish red. That is, hemolysin destroys the red cells, causing the release of hemoglobin (the pigment responsible for their red color). In the language of the laboratory, this annihilation of red cells is called hemolysis. On the other hand, if the rabbit serum is first *heated,* hemolysis does not occur, because heat destroys complement. In sum, red cells (antigen) and hemolysin (antibody) and complement interact to cause hemolysis.

Overnight various investigators perceived the diagnostic implications of these findings, and in 1906 the German bacteriologist, August Paul von Wassermann, and his fellow workers, Albert Neisser and Carl Bruck, devised the immortal *complement-fixation test* for syphilis, a revolutionary development in serology. Using an extract prepared from the liver of a stillborn syphilitic infant and an "indicator system" of sheep red cells and anti-sheep rabbit serum, these investigators demonstrated the presence of "diagnostic antibody" in the blood serum of syphilitic patients and its absence in normal serum. Briefly, appropriate and measured amounts of syphilitic antigen ("liver extract"), complement (from guinea pig

2. Called alexin by Bordet.

NEGATIVE WASSERMANN

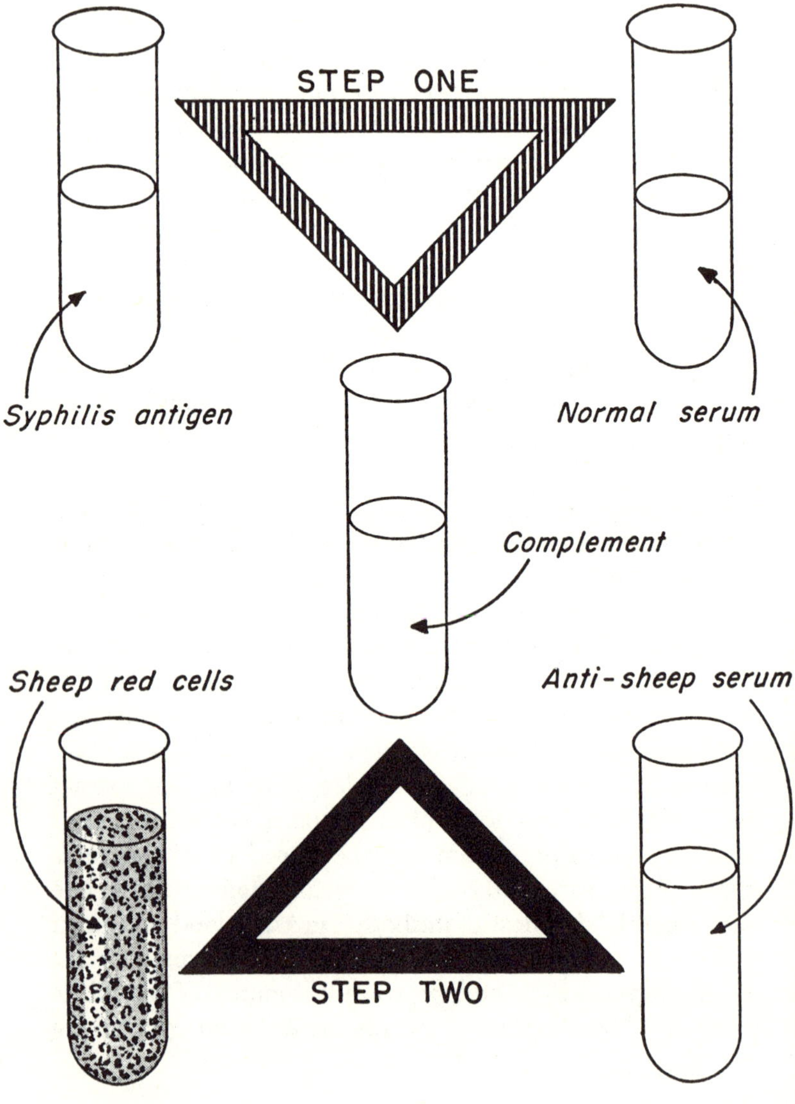

HEMOLYSIS

In the negative test, complement is *not* fixed in the first step, making it thus available to go on and effect hemolysis in the second step.

POSITIVE WASSERMANN

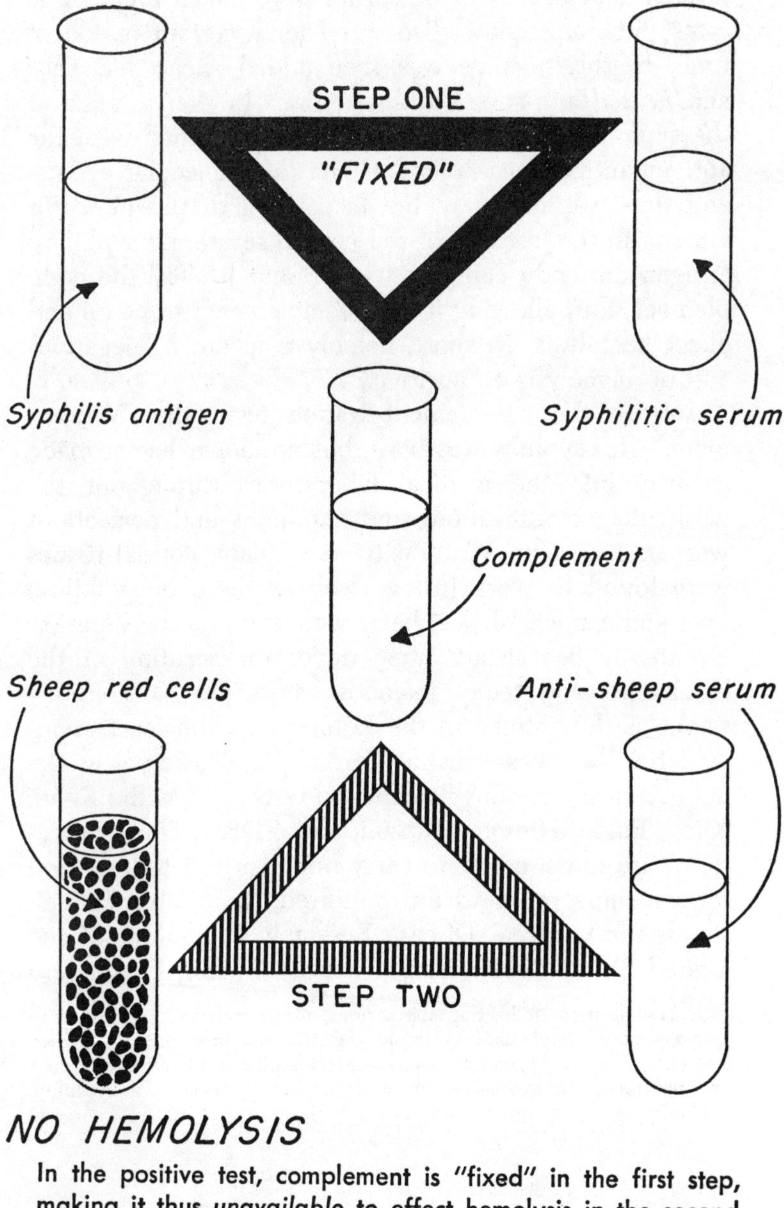

NO HEMOLYSIS

In the positive test, complement is "fixed" in the first step, making it thus *unavailable* to effect hemolysis in the second step.

serum), and *heated* blood serum were mixed together in a test tube and allowed to stand for a certain period of time; to this mixture was then added sheep red cells and *heated* anti-sheep rabbit serum.[3] In the instance of the syphilitic serum the complement combined with the antigen-antibody complex—an *invisible* molecular event—and thus was not available to react with the indicator system. In the instance of the normal serum, no syphilitic antigen–antibody complex was present to "fix" the complement, thus allowing it (the complement) to go on and effect hemolysis. In short, hemolysis meant a "negative" and no hemolysis a "positive."

And so the complement-fixation test (the "Wassermann") for syphilis was born, but no sooner had it made its way into the medical laboratories throughout the world than modifications and variations and perfections were on the scene. Water extracts of plain, normal tissues were found to work just as well as those of syphilitic liver and extracts of beef heart were found to be superior. Eventually beef heart came under the scrutiny of the biochemist and today its active principle—cardiolipin—serves as the antigen in the Kolmer test, the most popular latter day Wassermann. Cardiolipin also serves as the antigen in the various flocculation tests such as the Kahn, Kline, Eagle, Hinton, Mazzini, and VDRL. These procedures are much easier to carry out than the Kolmer and for screening purposes are preferred, the VDRL (which stands for Venereal Disease Research Laboratory of the United States Public Health Service) being by far and

3. The purpose in heating the serums, of course, was to make sure that the only complement available was the measured amount added, just enough to be "fixed" (in the event syphilitic antibody is present) and no more. An excess would result in hemolysis even if syphilitic antibody were present.

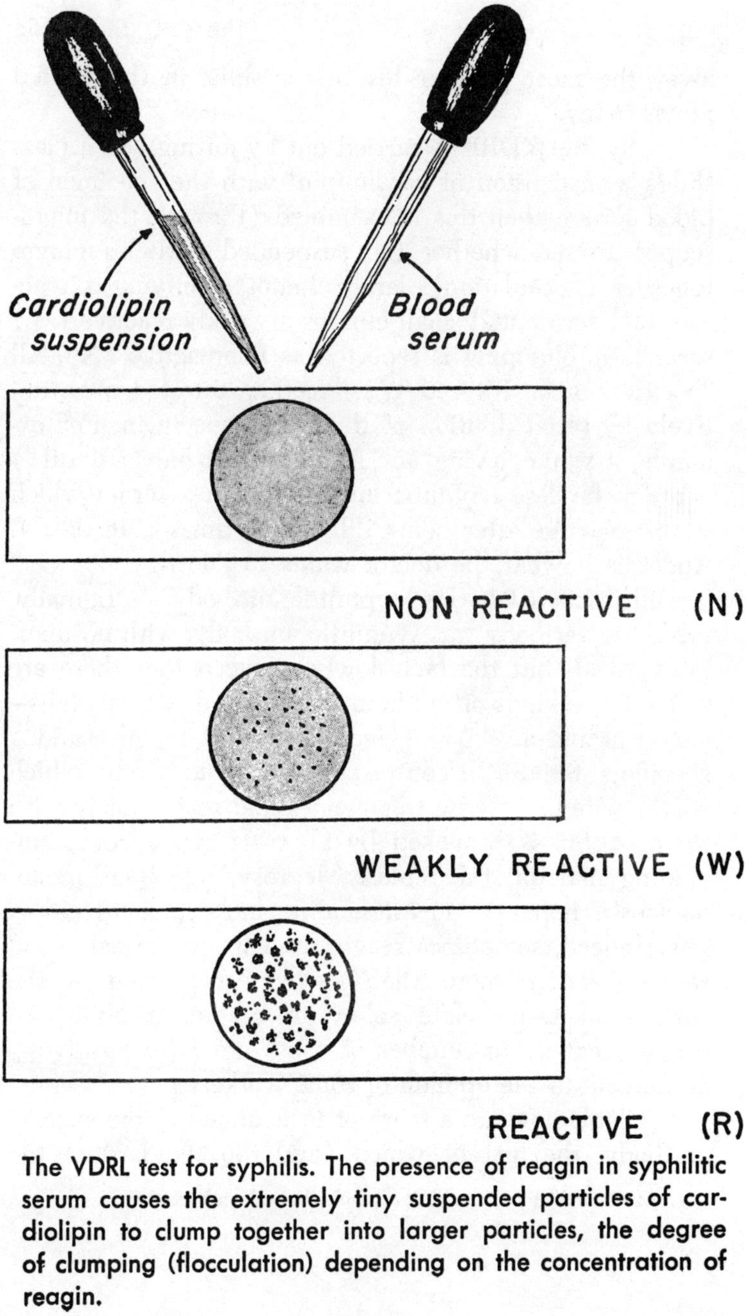

The VDRL test for syphilis. The presence of reagin in syphilitic serum causes the extremely tiny suspended particles of cardiolipin to clump together into larger particles, the degree of clumping (flocculation) depending on the concentration of reagin.

away the most popular test for syphilis in the United States today.

Briefly, the VDRL is carried out by mixing (on a glass slide) a suspension of cardiolipin[4] with the specimen of blood serum; then this is examined (through the microscope) to see whether the suspended particles clump together (flocculation), large clumps signifying a reactive (R) serum and small clumps a weakly reactive (W) serum. No clumping is reported as nonreactive (N). All "positives"—i.e., R's and W's—are then retested quantitatively by serial dilution of the serum specimen. For example, a serum giving an "R" undiluted only ("1 dil.") contains far less syphilitic antibody than a serum which is still reactive after being diluted 16 times ("16 dils."). And this is what the doctor wants to know.

And just what is this "syphilitic antibody"? Originally, syphilitic antibody was syphilitic antibody, with no questions asked; but the fact slowly surfaced that there are at least two kinds of antibodies associated with syphilis—a nonspecific antibody (given the name reagin) and a specific antibody. In contrast to specific antibody, which is stimulated solely by treponemes and reacts solely with them, reagin is provoked by all sorts of infections, including malaria, tuberculosis, leprosy, infectious mononucleosis, hepatitis, measles, and chickenpox, to cite a few. Indeed, sometimes reagin appears in normal blood serum. What is more, the "positives" registered by the cardiolipin tests relate solely to reagin, meaning, of course, that a fair number of these are *false* positives—20 percent in the opinion of some workers!

Available now are a score of tests aimed at the specific antibody, the first of which (and the standard of the

4. "Activated" by the addition of cholesterol and lecithin.

class) was introduced in 1949 by R. A. Nelson and M. M. Mayer. Appropriately called the "*Treponema pallidum* immobilization" (TPI) test, the procedure is carried out by adding complement and blood serum to live treponemes (obtained from the testicular lesions of infected rabbits) on a glass slide and watching to see (with the aid of the microscope) if these motile corkscrews grind to a halt. If they do, immobilizing–specific–antibody is present in the blood serum and the individual has a treponemal infection–almost always syphilis.

The TPI sounds easy on paper, but in practice the test is technically difficult, time consuming, and expensive. And this is because live treponemes are so terribly fragile. Consequently, the search was soon on for "dead treponemal tests," a quest which has resulted in some of the most fascinating maneuvers known to the diagnostic laboratory. The most valuable test of this kind to date is FTA-ABS, which stands for "Fluorescent Treponemal Antibody-Absorption." The basic procedure is this: A drop or two of a suspension of live pathogenic treponemes is placed on a glass slide and the slide heated to kill them and stick ("fix") them to the glass. Next the patient's blood serum is mixed with an extract of nonpathogenic treponemes (Reiter strain) to absorb any and all antibodies *except* those specific to *Treponema pallidum*, the purged serum then being applied to the slide. Now, if specific antibodies are indeed present they will attach to the fixed treponemes, and in order to prove or disprove it fluorescein-tagged "antihuman antibody" (prepared from the blood of animals immunized against human antibody) is next applied. The slide is then rinsed and examined through the ultraviolet microscope. *Glowing* treponemes signal a positive test. That is, the pa-

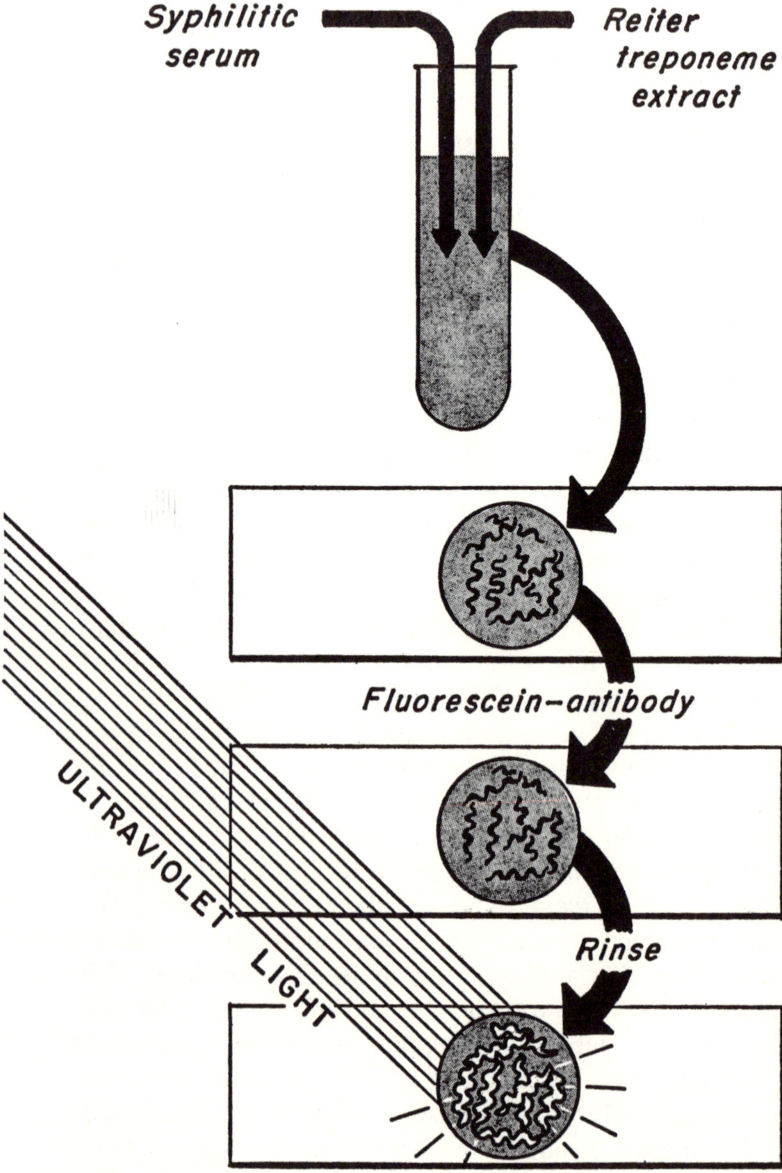

The FTA-ABS test, showing the basic steps. In "this instance" the test is positive.

tient's treponemal antibody has attached to the treponemes and the fluorescein-tagged antibody has in turn attached to the treponemal antibody. In the absence of treponemal antibody (normal blood serum) there is nothing for the fluorescein-tagged antibody to attach to and it is rinsed away. Thus, the treponemes do not glow—a negative test.

To return to the reagin tests, these possess phenomenal sensitivity and the speedy versions, such as the VDRL, are well suited to routine screening. Also, they are the tests of choice in monitoring the response to treatment, a dropping reagin titer (concentration) signaling the desired response. Indeed, a negative VDRL signals a cure. Further, a dropping reagin titer in the newborn usually indicates a passive transfer of that antibody from the mother, whereas a *rising* titer usually means congenital syphilis. By contrast, specific or treponemal antibody, once present, persists for life with or without treatment. (Early treatment prevents the appearance of both antibodies.) Thus, these tests, the FTA-ABS and others, are used mostly as confirmatory tools in problem cases, namely where nothing points to syphilis except a positive Kolmer, VDRL or what have you. A negative FTA-ABS in the face of a reactive VDRL points to a classic false positive.

False positives, it almost goes without saying, also arise from technical error, which more or less accounts for the expression "biological" false positive. For instance, if a patient with hepatitis—not syphilis—is, let us say, "VDRL positive" there is a biological reason—namely, a virus. On the other hand, the reason for a positive on *normal* blood relates to some technical difficulty. Perhaps one might characterize this event as a "true" false positive. And, too, there is the matter of false negatives, serological tests in general giving 80 to 90 percent positives with *known* syphilitic specimens. The presence of insufficient reagin accounts for many false negatives and this obtains in several phases of the disease, especially in early primary syphilis (where a *positive* test does not develop until about a month *after* infection) and late latent syphilis. Again, in neurosyphilis, notably tabes dorsalis, the serology may be negative in nearly half the cases.

Let us now turn to the laboratory consideration of the cerebrospinal fluid, the crystal clear fluid which bathes the spinal cord and fills the spaces (ventricles) within the brain. This fluid derives from the blood serum and has about the same chemical profile save for its low content of protein. Roughly speaking "cerebrospinal tests" fall within the purview of serology, but strictly speaking they compose a body of information often well beyond the reach of blood serum. Cerebrospinal fluid affords the only means of diagnosing neurosyphilis accurately and evaluating its treatment. And a diagnosis of latent syphilis cannot be made unless asymptomatic neurosyphilis is excluded by negative findings. A positive Kolmer or VDRL (carried out in the same manner as on blood serum) practically always indicates nervous system involvement. Additionally, the number of lymphocytes (a type of white cell) and amount of protein indicate the degree of neurosyphilis and the effectiveness of treatment. Usually the lymphocyte count returns to normal first, followed by a drop in protein. As no mere rule of thumb, then, the cerebrospinal fluid should be examined and studied in *every* case of syphilis.

In closing, let us not forsake the patient with his signs

and symptoms—or lack of them—for the test tube. Clearly, all these serological tests are wonderful and fascinating and indispensable, but they must always be viewed and interpreted in the context of the total picture. Also, we must not forsake *Treponema pallidum,* for absolutely nothing supersedes a "positive darkfield" in the diagnosis of syphilis.

5
Treatment, Yesterday

Among the hundreds of thousands of remedies and medicaments which have graced the apothecary shelf, few present a past charged with as many trials and tribulations as mercury. Since time immemorial this liquid metal ("quicksilver") and its compounds have been used and misused for every conceivable illness and ailment known to man and beast. By the 16th century mercury had come into general use as an antisyphilitic throughout the civilized world, and then in a most undulating fashion made its way to the mid 1940s—to penicillin. From the first some swore by it and others against it, and for excellent reason on both sides. Or, to put it directly, mercury poisoned and killed treponemes all right, but it also poisoned and upon occasion killed the patient. In the context of syphilology, mercury poisoning was a way of life, and not uncommonly among the unknowing taken to be a phase of the tertiary stage. And so the old saying, something to the effect that "a night with Venus meant the rest of your days with Mercury," was clearly an accurate appraisal of the situation. Be that as it may, mercury, to repeat, did kill treponemes and with the possible exception of potassium iodide (which had some therapeutic value) it was the only "truly efficacious" remedy available up until Germany's Paul Ehrlich came along with his "magic bullet" in the year 1909.

As usual in the workings of history, the events leading up to Ehrlich's discovery were evolutionary in the true sense of the word. In 1863, Bechamp, in search for a drug against African sleeping sickness, synthesized an arsenical known to chemistry as sodium arsanilate and to medicine as atoxyl. It proved moderately successful. Medical investigators at large then began looking around for other obliging parasites, a quest which bore fruit many years later when the German bacteriologist Paul Uhlenhuth demonstrated atoxyl's effectiveness in spirillosis (a fatal spirochete infection of chickens and other fowl). This exciting development led to the drug's use in syphilis. And the results were both good and bad; that is, it killed the spirochetes, but poisoned the patient at the needed dosage—mercury all over again. Ehrlich upon getting wind of this was nonetheless optimistic and set out to prove his pet theory that for every infection the chemist can come up with a chemical which will smite the parasite and spare the host.

Thus began one of those tales medicine so much likes to tell—a man with a dream looking for a golden remedy to cure a dread disease. Arsenical after arsenical was synthesized and tested, the idea being to package an atom or two of spirocheticidal arsenic in a harmless molecular sac. Finally, in 1909, after the 606th try, Ehrlich and his co-worker Sachachiro Hata came upon the magical yellowish powder arsphenamine. The man on the street, and most particularly the man with syphilis, would come to know it as Salvarsan or "606." Relative to mercury arsphenamine was indeed a wonder drug—a "magic bullet"—and became the mainstay in the management of syphilis up until penicillin. But in an absolute sense, needless to say, the yellow chemical left much to be desired. A cure required months and months of injections, and worst of all, of course, the stuff commonly proved toxic in the long drawn out case. Ehrlich pushed himself to the very limit to perfect the drug, but the best he could do—the best he could synthesize—was neoarsphenamine (compound "914"). Though neutral and very soluble in water and thus a little easier to handle than "606" pharmaceutically, it proved no more effective therapeutically.

Meanwhile a number of workers were looking into the therapeutic possibilities of bismuth (a metal similar chemically to mercury) and in 1922 the Rumanian bacteriologist Constantin Levaditi reported favorable results in 200 cases of syphilis. The metal (or rather its compounds) proved less effective than the mercurials and arsenicals, but on the other hand it was much less toxic. This, of course, was no small virtue and before long and up until the advent of penicillin the "treatment of choice" in the typical case of the disease was the alternate use of arsenicals and so-called "heavy metals" (that is, bismuth and mercury). The multiple attack did a good job in getting rid of the treponemes and at the same time was moderately kind to the host. It usually cured early syphilis.

But the late stages of the disease were often refractory to any kind of chemical attack, and this was especially true in the more severe forms of neurosyphilis. Consequently, other therapeutic approaches were probed and in 1917 the Viennese psychiatrist, Julius von Wagner-Jauregg, reported a good number of cures in psychotic syphilitics using "malarial injections." The salutary effects

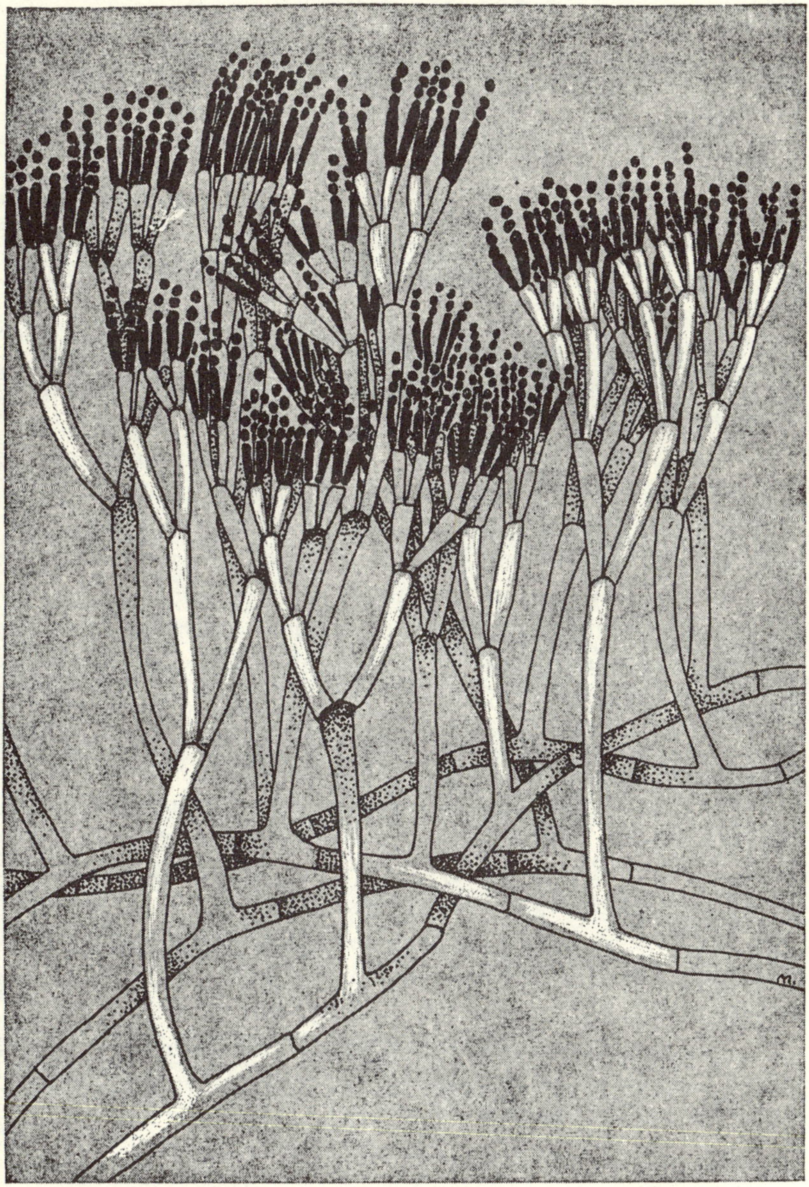

Penicillium notatum, the mold which produces penicillin (expanded 1,200x).

of fever in such cases had been appreciated for some time, and so to induce it artificially under controlled conditions was the height of genius. In brief the treatment was carried out by injecting the malarial parasite *Plasmodium vivax* and then terminating the infection (malaria!) with quinine. Perfection in this area came with the advent of less drastic measures and in this country the Kettering electronic cabinet became the device of choice.

Wagner-Jauregg received the Nobel Prize in 1927, just one year before a Scottish bacteriologist by the name of Alexander Fleming took note of the destructive action of the greenish mold *Penicillium notatum* against a certain tribe of disease-producing streptococci. Others had seen this, too, but no one *noted it!* Quite apparently this was a glaring example of antibiosis (or "life against life"), that is, mold against bacterium. More particularly, reasoned Fleming, the mold manufactured an antibiotic substance—an antibiotic he very appropriately christened penicillin.

Great events not infrequently get off to a slow start, and such was the case here. The years passed and not until Ernst Chain, a German pathologist, and Howard Florey, an English pathologist, came along in the late 1930s did the wheels of science turn in a practical way. First, Chain and Florey confirmed Fleming's phenomenon and then went on to actually isolate the magical chemical. And when enough of it was available to make its way to the bedside miracles started to happen. In 1943 John Mahoney, a New York physician, added the finishing touch—to wit, a shot or two of penicillin cured syphilis! And so, therapeutically anyway, the syphilis story is a matter of "before" and "after" penicillin.

6
Penicillin

The management of syphilis centers upon the use of penicillin to kill the invader and "follow-up" serology to monitor the response. The goal is a "biologic cure"—the complete eradication of *all* treponemes. Dosage, details of follow-up, and prognosis relate to what we might call the three "therapeutic phases" of the disease—*early, late latent,* and *late*. Early—or "infectious syphilis"—covers the first and second stages and the *early* latent period. Late latent is exactly what it says, and "late" refers to tertiary syphilis. In regard to the kind of penicillin used—dozens are available—the long-acting versions are preferred with PAM (procaine penicillin G with 2 percent aluminum monostearate) and benzathine penicillin G (Bicillin) being favorites, especially the latter. When penicillin cannot be tolerated by reason of hypersensitivity, substitute antibiotics, such as erythromycin and the "tetracyclines," are used, but sometimes with less effectiveness.

The highlights in the handling of a typical case of early syphilis at a typical clinic run about as follows: On "day one" the doctor injects 2.4 million units of Bicillin—1.2 million deep into each buttock. And this is about it as far as drugs are concerned. From then on it is a wait and see affair. In about six hours (following the shot) the chancre—*if* present—gets puffy, the satellite buboes—*if* present—enlarge, and the rash—*if* present—intensifies, a disappearing rash commonly returning to full bloom. The temperature jumps up, sometimes to 103° or 104°F. This pharmacologic paradox, first noted by two German dermatologists, Adolph Jarisch and Karl Herxheimer, and known to medicine as the Jarisch-Herxheimer reaction, attests to the *efficacy* of the medication. Although there is no unanimous agreement on the microbial and biochemical details, the usual explanation relates to the release of toxic materials from the carcasses of the slaughtered treponemes. The reaction lasts two or three hours. Within 24 hours of the injection, the lesions show onset of resolution and the treponemes are no longer demonstrable! Within seven to ten days the lesions are all but healed!! The serology at this time is positive but gradually works its way to negative in three or four months. If still negative at twelve months and there are no signs or symptoms the patient is cured.

Generally speaking biologic cures are effected in about 90 percent of early syphilitics who receive *one* course of treatment and in a substantial proportion of those who must be retreated. When treatment is instituted in *early* early syphilis—that is, before the blood serum goes positive—the figure is probably closer to 98 percent. A very few fail to become "seronegative" and the consensus here is that if the reagin is low and if there is no clinical evidence of the disease, then these patients may be safely followed without further treatment.

And finally there is the rather uncommon phenomenon of relapsing, or the rebirth of the disease in the wake of "successful treatment." Paradoxically, the situation may prove more severe than in the course of relapsing *untreated* syphilis, especially in regard to complications associated with the eye and nervous system. Additionally, these people may not consider their "new condition" venereal and thus become a real health hazard. Undoubtedly a good number of such therapeutic failures stem from reinfection, a much greater possibility now than in the old "606 days" because once the treponemes are eradicated the body is no longer immune to infection.

Late latent syphilis presents a dilemma of sorts because once *true* latency is established it is quite probable that therapy is not needed. Moreover, the treponemes at this period of the infection are not believed to be particularly sensitive to penicillin. Be that as it may, latent syphilis can and does evolve into late, or tertiary, syphilis, and for this reason and this reason alone the patient is given penicillin. The dose is usually the same as in early syphilis—that is, 1.2 million units (of Bicillin) deep into each buttock. But *before* this is given the cerebrospinal fluid is examined to confirm the diagnosis. If it is negative, we shall recall, the patient is indeed in latency; if it is positive the patient has late, or tertiary, syphilis.

Inasmuch as latency presents no signs and symptoms the effect of penicillin on the course of the disease can only be ascertained by following the patient throughout his entire life, a state of affairs which restricts an evaluation. The best we can do, then, is to extrapolate the results in other forms of syphilis, and when this is done the prognosis appears most favorable. The *Cecil-Loeb Textbook of Medicine* states: "A reasonable prediction would be that less than 2 percent of patients with late latent syphilis who are properly treated will subsequently develop serious manifestations of late syphilis." Interestingly, the serology not uncommonly fails to parallel or reflect the clinical outlook. Reagin drops very slowly and treponemal immobilizing antibody does not reverse itself at all. This failure to return to normal—this *seroresistance* to penicillin—is a cardinal phenomenon of "latent therapy" and a perennial source of *misunderstanding* among the laity: come hell or high water, a "positive Wassermann" means syphilis and so on. . . . The reader well knows by now that syphilis always means reagin, but reagin by no means always means syphilis. In short, the seroresistance of late latent syphilis is the lingering smoke of an extinguished fire. Further water—further penicillin—does not "put the smoke out."

By and large *late* syphilis calls for more penicillin and more follow-up; for instance, 9 million units (as Bicillin) and physical and serologic check-ups at three- and six-month intervals during the first and second years, respectively. In the benign version of the stage, when the cardiovascular and nervous systems are not involved, the prognosis is good to excellent. Within the first few days following the first shot the patient starts to feel much better and the lesions—the gummas—start to heal, and in a matter of weeks or months, depending upon the size and number of gummas, the patient is clinically cured. Serum reagin drops somewhat, but typically lingers on and on, as does the immobilizing antibody.

The outlook in neurosyphilis runs from excellent to hopeless. Clearly, nothing can be done to redeem damaged tissue. In *asymptomatic* neurosyphilis—where the only sign is a "positive" cerebrospinal fluid—immediate therapy can prevent the development of the various *symptomatic* forms of the involvement. Periodic examination of the cerebrospinal fluid is especially critical here, a negative test signifying "a cure." *Meningeal* neurosyphilis responds, often dramatically, to treatment in two or three days, but the ultimate outcome is rather unpredictable. In the face of brain damage, paralysis, severe mental impairment or both are quite possible. *Vascular* neurosyphilis responds much much less effectively and the prognosis is generally poor. *Tabes dorsalis* responds better than one might expect, just about all patients showing some improvement. And in regard to syphilitic insanity, the best penicillin can do is to impede further deterioration of mind and body. Because in these patients the Jarisch-Herxheimer reaction can trigger startling repercussions, including convulsion, hospitalization is a must. A few specialists, incidentally, augment their penicillin shots with fever therapy using "therapeutic malaria," one regimen calling for 40 hours of temperatures over 104°F.

Pregnant syphilitic women are treated like anyone else —but faster. To be on the safe side—and the only side as far as syphilis is concerned—all former patients should have monthly serologic tests throughout pregnancy. And in the event of *doubt* regarding diagnosis or adequacy of previous management, retreatment is the order of the day.

Congenital syphilis responds dramatically to penicillin and complete cures are the rule when the infection is caught in the perennial "nip in the bud" stage. Afflicted youngsters under two years of age are usually cured in one year, and even in late congenital syphilis (12 years or older) the prognosis is good provided there is no real damage at the commencement of treatment. Save for the adjunctive use of corticosteroids when the treponemes attack the eye (interstitial keratitis) a shot of Bicillin, deep into each buttock, does the trick.

7
Preventives

Penicillin—Paul Erhlich's dream come true—can cure syphilis, and penicillin can control syphilis; but here the "magic bullet" is of greater caliber than the one the doctor shoots into the buttock. You certainly cannot control syphilis unless you sight the target, unless you zero in on the disease in progress or the disease about to be. This—this greater caliber—means prompt diagnosis and the immediate gathering together of all sexual partners—"contacts"—through "casefinding." A couple of shots of Bicillin cures early, infectious, syphilis. A couple of shots of Bicillin prevents syphilis in fresh contacts. And the fresh contact is the most lethal contact because he or she is sign and symptom free, a silent and most excellent purveyor of *Treponema pallidum.* In one classic study in a small southern town a 14-year-old girl passed the disease on to her baby and boyfriend, who in turn passed it on to three other teenagers, who in turn passed it on to seven boys. And so on. All told, 23 cases emerged through casefinding and were successfully treated.

At every turn routine blood tests must be instituted to identify the disease in the sleeping phases, and there is no reason in the world why a VDRL cannot be performed right along with any other test. Also, the U. S. Public Health Service recommends that a serologic test be made in pregnancy at the patient's first visit to the doctor and at intervals thereafter. Proper treatment of the syphilitic mother before the breakdown in the placenta of Langhan's layer (which occurs about the 17th week after conception) will totally prevent the invasion of the fetus by treponemes. All of this means astronomical testing, especially when we consider the 38 million tests for syphilis already being performed annually in the United States. In short, there is a great need for automation and to meet this challenge a number of laboratories are doing amazing things. The FTA-ABS has been automated and a whole series of reagin procedures, euphoniously labeled "ART" (for Automated Reagin Test), are now available.

The epitome of prophylaxis, of course, is vaccination and for years investigators all over the world have tried to perfect a vaccine against syphilis. One investigative approach has been the use of killed *Treponema pallida.* In a recent experiment carried out in Poland, such a vaccine inoculated into rabbits prevented the development of syphilitic lesions when "challenged" by live treponemes. And in this country an exciting investigation is underway at the U. S. Public Health Service's Venereal Disease Research Center in Atlanta. In 1968 three male chimpanzees were inoculated at multiple sites with infective material from two untreated patients with pinta, a rather mild skin disease caused by *Treponema carateum.* All three chimps have developed pinta and once certain technical matters are attended to they will be challenged with *Treponema pallidum* to ascertain if pinta does indeed induce immunity to syphilis. And this is certainly not unreasonable thinking. Just about every person reading this sentence is immune to smallpox as a consequence of a prior artificial infection with vaccinia. That is to say, "smallpox vaccine" contains the *live* virus of vaccinia (a very mild infection in man), the latter stimulating the body to produce antibodies against *both* diseases. Who knows, perhaps one day a shot of domesticated *Treponema carateum* will be the answer to the great pox.

Meanwhile we must put to work all the forces now available—serology, casefinding, prompt treatment, and education. And yes, condoms and soap and water.

GONORRHEA

8
Backgrounds

Gonorrhea is the most common venereal disease of universal stature. Like syphilis, its incidence is highest in the cities, among the underprivileged, among Blacks, and in males. In the United States the disease has assumed a rollercoaster prevalence since 1940, when there were 175,841 *reported* cases (133.8 per 100,000 population). By 1947 it had jumped to 400,639 cases (284.2 per 100,000) and then, thanks to penicillin, in 1957 the *rate* fell to an all time low of 129 per 100,000 (216,476 cases). But quite apparently penicillin cannot win V.D. wars single-handedly, because the 1970 rate hit the statistic of 285.2 per 100,000—a staggering 573,200 reported cases! The actual prevalence is estimated by the Venereal Disease Branch of the United States Public Health Service to be at least two million cases!!

Historically and otherwise, etymologically for instance, gonorrhea antedates syphilis. Well known to the ancients, it was first named by none other than the celebrated Greek physician Galen (130–200 A.D.), or Claudius Galenus, as he was known in Rome. *Gono-*, in Greek, refers to semen, and *rhein* means "to flow;" so apparently what Galen had in mind was something to do with the *ab-*

normal flow of semen. But an ejaculation, needless to say, is a far cry from a discharge, so actually *blenorrhea,* the other medical expression for the infection, is closer to the mark, meaning as it does (in Greek) "the flow of mucus" —pussy (*pus i!*) mucus, that is. Decades ago the public at large reluctantly called it "clap" even in such wholesome publications as "The Household Physician" and the "Century Book of Health."

By way of review, the Swiss alchemist Phillipus Aureolus Bombastus Paracelsus von Hohenheim (1493–1541) "Paracelsus" for short (although the third name in is more appropriate), came up with the idea that gonorrhea was a prelude to syphilis and in 1767 England's famed surgeon John Hunter "proved it." French physician Philippe Ricord finally put the record straight in 1838 (pun not necessarily intended). . . . And now to fill out the story: in 1879 the German physician Albert Neisser called attention to the "constant presence of a peculiar coccus" (roundish microbe) in gonorrheal pus, and in 1885 a Doctor Bumm demonstrated its (the microbe's) etiologic relationship to gonorrhea by inoculating human volunteers. Over the years Neisser's "peculiar coccus" has been given a variety of scientific names, but today the only one recognized by all authorities is *Neisseria gonorrhoeae.* Among doctors and nurses it is referred to colloquially as "the gonococcus."

Neisseria gonorrhoeae is actually what the bacteriologist calls a diplococcus, that is, a bacterium with roundish cells (cocci) typically occurring *in pairs.* As a point of reference, staphylococci ("staph") occur in grapelike bunches and streptococci ("strep") occur in chains. Gonococci are small as bacteria go, a dozen or more "pairs" often crowding into a *single* white blood cell—and it takes

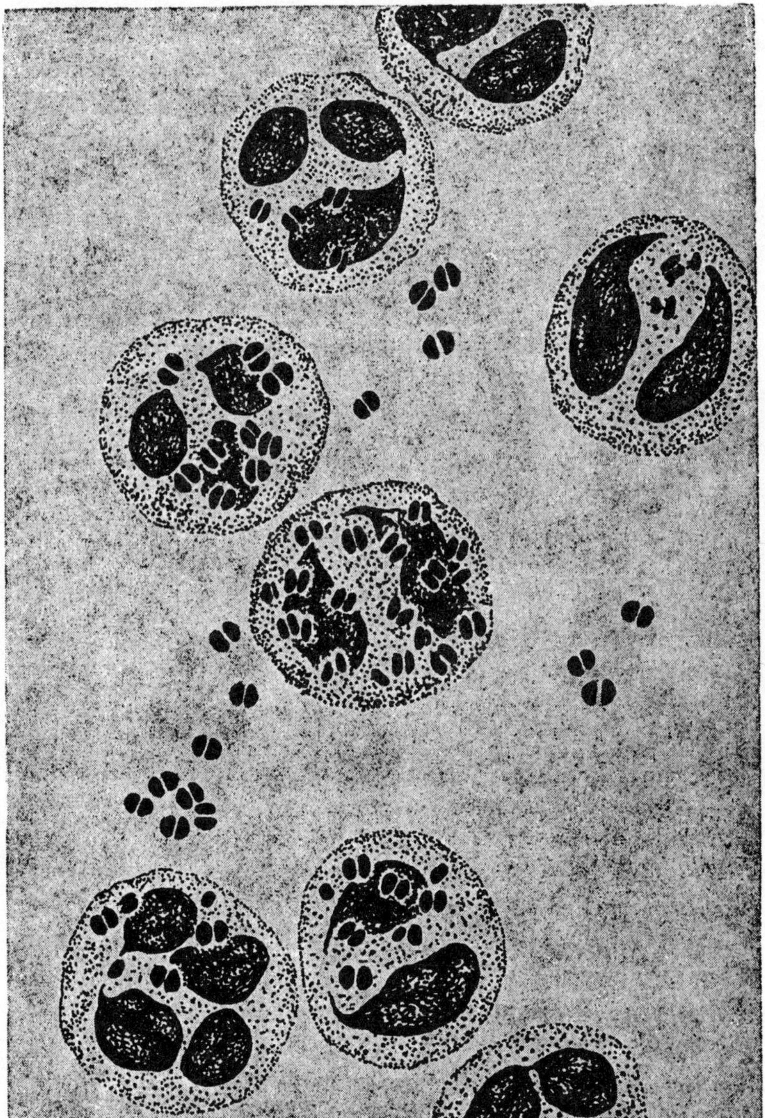

Neisseria gonorrhoeae in pus, showing gonococci both within and outside the large leukocytes ("pus cells"). Note their typical coffee-bean shape and arrangement in pairs (expanded 3,000x).

about 2,000 white cells to span an inch! Further, and characteristically, these cocci possess flattened sides in juxtaposition, stained preparations reminding one of coffee beans.

Physiologically, the gonococcus is at once frail and fussy. Only one situation really and truly suits it and that's *human* mucous membranes. The slightest chemical or physical influence can come along and cause immediate death. Weak disinfectants, moderately high temperatures, drying, and supersonic sound waves, to mention a few possibilities, easily do the trick. And, too, the gonococcus does not even like ordinary air, much preferring an atmosphere charged with 10 percent carbon dioxide. Its favorite temperature is 95°F. and its favorite food is the blood pigment hemoglobin. . . . Above all, *Neisseria gonorrhoeae* does not like toilet seats!

9
The Disease

The gonococcus readily attacks mucous membranes and this well explains its venereal proclivities. Man and man alone is its only natural target and not until 1970 did anyone succeed in producing *artificial* gonorrhea in animals. This was done at the government's famed Venereal Disease Research Laboratory in Atlanta, where two male chimpanzees were inoculated urethrally with active pus from a patient at a local clinic. Both chimps developed a typical case of gonorrhea and one developed gonorrheal conjunctivitis via autoinoculation. And to really clinch this exciting development, a third chimp was infected by urethral exudate from these two animals. Now for the first time researchers have at their disposal a living laboratory model to study the disease under controlled conditions. Exciting advancements—for example, new serologic blood tests—are already in the pilot stage.

The mechanism by which the gonococcus effects its mischief is still not understood, notwithstanding years and years of laboratory interest and effort. Many virulent bacteria produce potent poisons called *exo*toxins, but this is not the case here. Conceivably, disintegrating dead gonococcal cells liberate noxious substances called endotoxins. Be that as it may, the organism thrives and multiplies, leaving in its wake burning disheveled tissue and abundant pus.

The infected partner infects the noninfected partner by introducing a "dose" of gonococci into the fluid products of the sexual act. That is to say, they, the gonococci, are massaged and washed into the urethral orifice in a most efficient manner. The usual incubation period—the time between contact and the first signs and symptoms of the invasion—runs between three and nine days. In the male, in the typical case, the first signs are burning on urination and the appearance of a pussy discharge. Too, the urethral orifice is usually inflamed and puffy. The infection then works its way upward and backward through the urethra and shortly incites real trouble in the prostate gland and seminal vesicles, the former (prostatitis) squeezing the urethra and causing urinary retention and the latter causing fever and pain. Further advancement of the infection into the seminal duct leads to inflammation of the epididymis, the sperm reservoir attached to the upper surface of the testicle. Generally, the entire testicle is swollen and exquisitely painful and tender. Following successful treatment these signs and symptoms gradually subside, but there may be important and serious complications as we shall see in a moment.

Gonorrhea in the female is a pathologic enigma and the unwary reader can be easily misled even by some of the better medical texts. In point of fact the *early* stages of the disease *usually* do not appear, and on good authority perhaps nine out of ten victims *may* be completely without signs and symptoms! This well explains the "more common occurrence" in the male. Moreover, it well explains why the disease is so difficult to control. When

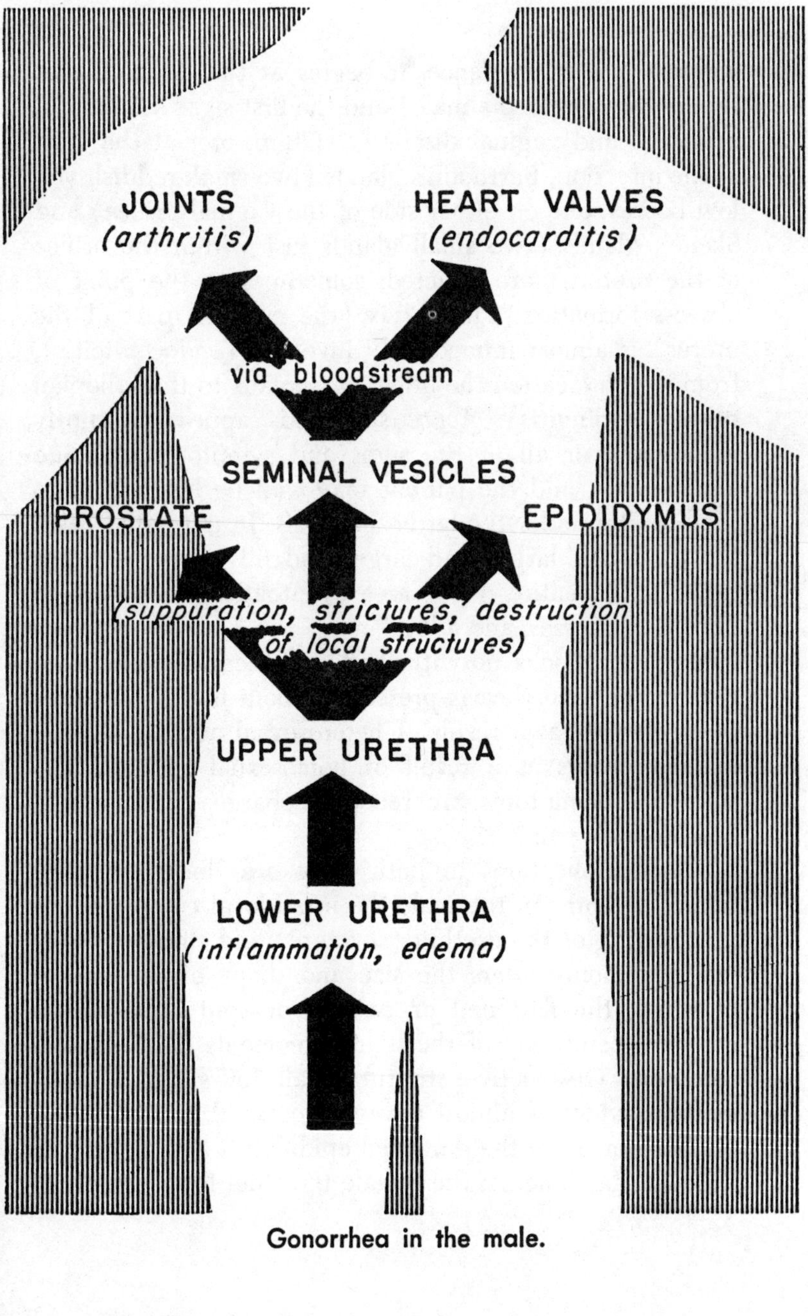

Gonorrhea in the male.

gonorrhea *is* in evidence, it begins at the beginning of the urethra (as in the male) and the first signs are painful urination and vaginal discharge. Often, too, at the start of the infection, Bartholin's glands (two small reddish yellow bodies, one on either side of the vaginal orifice) and Skene's glands (two small glands just within the orifice of the urethra) are afflicted, sometimes to the point of abscess formation. The cervix (the necklike part of the uterus) is almost immediately involved (endocervicitis), from which location the infection spreads to the fallopian tubes (salpingitis). *Acute* salpingitis appears abruptly with many or all of the signs and symptoms of acute appendicitis, and the patient may well be hustled off to the hospital under the latter diagnosis. In untreated cases the tubes get larger and larger and fill with pus ("pus tubes"), the entire pelvic area eventually giving way to fibrosis, abscesses, and adhesions.

Many textbooks notwithstanding, recent data indicate that *rectal* gonorrhea is present in about half of all cases in the female as a result of heterosexual activity. In the male it occurs as a result of homosexual activity. The signs and symptoms are rectal discharge, burning and considerable pain.

The complications in both sexes are "local" or "systemic" or both. In the male the usual local complications are scarring of the urethra (stricture) and sterility. Stricture commonly alters the size and shape of the stream of urine, the flattened or twisted or split stream conceivably being one of the lighter moments of diagnostic medicine. Obstructive strictures call for surgical intervention, which is almost always successful. Sterility generally stems from the damaged epididymis and about this little can be done. In the female the chief local complica-

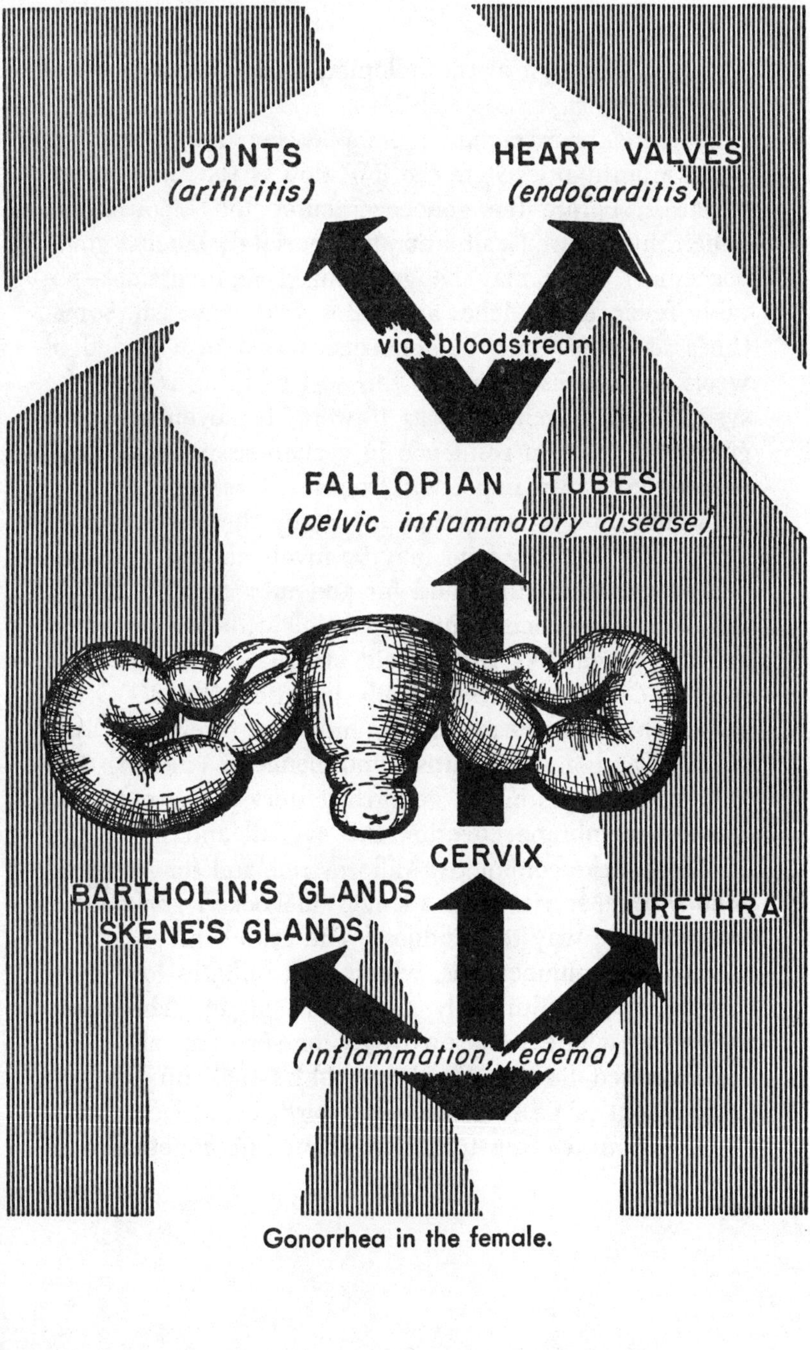

Gonorrhea in the female.

tion is obstruction of the fallopian tubes and consequent sterility.

Systemic, or extragenital, complications are rarer today because antibiotics stem the infection at the "local level" —that is, before the gonococci enter the bloodstream. When this occurs (a situation appropriately labeled gonococcemia) there may be generalized repercussions—notably fever, chills, aches and pains, and skin rash. Sometimes repeated bouts of gonococcemia span a period of weeks or months. Actually, this sort of thing is only the systemic dress rehearsal, as it were, for eventually the gonococci take up residence in certain tissues and there proceed to cause important trouble. "Site number one" is the joint, or rather, *joints*, especially the knees, wrists, and ankles. But any joint may be involved, and in a sudden sharp, fluctuating, and hit and miss fashion—hence, the expression "acute migratory polyarthritis." More or less it is much like rheumatoid arthritis, and sometimes the two conditions are clinically indistinguishable. Other sites include the heart valves, and very rarely the liver (hepatitis), bones (myelitis), and meninges (meningitis).

A special topic in the gonorrhea story is the eye. The delicate membrane covering the eyeball and lining the lids—called the conjunctiva—affords rich soil for *Neisseria gonorrhoeae*, so rich that a single unchecked gonococcus can pave the way to blindness! The initial infection is a fulminating conjunctivitis, which then radiates to deeper structures and ultimately the entire organ. The adult patient may infect his own eyes or someone else's via contaminated fingers. Newborn babies pick up the eye involvement in passing through a birth canal laden with gonococci. And often forgotten about but nonetheless a distinct possibility is the fact that a child (or adult) with gonorrheal conjunctivitis may infect its genitals.

Older textbooks and a sprinkling of noninitiated new ones make much to do about gonorrheal vulvovaginitis among little girls, and for good reason. Whereas the adult vulva (external genital organs) and vagina are lined with a rather resistant membrane, the prepuberty structure amounts to little more than a mucous membrane, like the one lining the urethra in all age groups. Thus, childhood vulvovaginitis—often epidemic among institutionalized children—was placed at the door of the gonococcus (contaminated toilet seats again!). Today we know there are dozens of different kinds of pathogens, all omnipresent, which attack the adolescent vulva and vagina, and some of them look exactly like *Neisseria gonorrhoeae*. Indeed, this is the origin of the myth. To be sure, gonorrheal vulvovaginitis does occur in little girls but when it does the cause is almost always venereal!

10
Tests

One particular trip to the bathroom sent Mr. A to the doctor, and for excellent reason. There was intense burning on urination, heralded by a creamy ooze. At the doctor's office Mr. A managed to massage forth a few drops of specimen and post haste this was sent to the laboratory for bacteriologic scrutiny. And sent along too was a note reading "Probable gonorrhea." Mr. A did mention, incidentally, a certain Miss B, and so forth.

The laboratory people first prepare "smears" and "streak plates," to use the technical vernacular. A smear is made by spreading—"smearing"—the specimen (in this case pus) across a spotlessly clean glass slide and then staining it to visualize and accentuate any microorganisms. The classic staining procedure and the one used here is the "gram stain," named after its Danish originator Hans Christian Gram. In brief—and in the following *order*—the smear is: stained with crystal violet; treated with iodine solution; rinsed in alcohol; counterstained with safranin; and rinsed in water. Some bacterial cells "react" with crystal violet and iodine in such a way that the color becomes "fixed and fast" and resistant to alcohol. Other bacteria *do not* fix the crystal violet-iodine com-

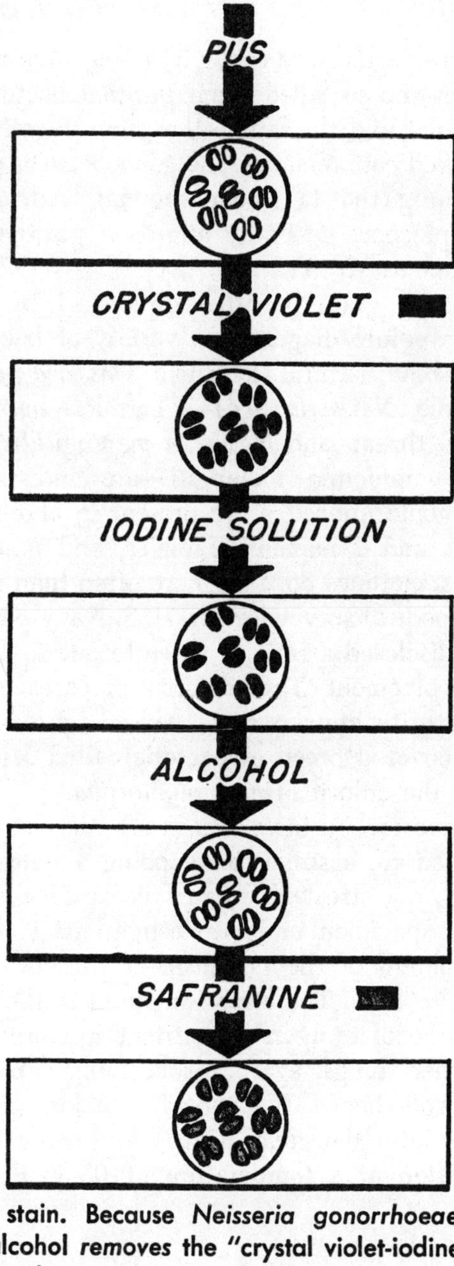

The gram stain. Because *Neisseria gonorrhoeae* is gram-negative, alcohol *removes* the "crystal violet-iodine complex" thus allowing the gonococci to take the counterstain, safranine.

plex and are decolorized easily by the alcohol rinse. Thus, the former—the so-called gram *positive* bacteria—remain blue or violet and the latter—the gram *negative* bacteria—take the red counterstain. The gonococcus is gram *negative,* meaning that a smear showing red, coffee-bean shaped diplococci generally affords a positive diagnosis in cases such as Mr. A's.

But finding gram negative diplococci by no means spells an absolute diagnosis. A variety of bacteria—some harmless, some harmful—look like *Neisseria gonorrhoeae.* For example, *Neisseria sicca*—a harmless habitué of the mouth and throat—and *Neisseria meningitidis*—the cause of deadly epidemic meningitis—are indistinguishable. Nonpathogenic imposters are present in about 3 percent of females and 2 percent of males, and nongonococcal urethritis sometimes pops up more often than gonococcal! A recent medical survey among U. S. Navy personnel, for instance, disclosed a ratio of three to one in favor of the former involvement. The majority of cases of nongonococcal urethritis appears to be caused by a relatively recently discovered breed of bacteria called *Mimeae,* most especially the culprit *Mima polymorpha.*

This impostor business brings up the "streak plates" just referred to, a streak plate being a culture medium inoculated, or "streaked," across its surface with a tiny bit of the specimen under investigation. The idea is to culture enough of the organism—if present—to perform *confirmatory* tests. The classic medium in the instance at hand is "chocolate agar," a nutrient mixture containing, among other things, agar (a solidifying substance) and heated blood—hence, the chocolate color. (Fresh blood tends to inhibit the gonococcus.) Following a day or so of incubation at a temperature of 95-96°F and in an atmosphere of 10 percent carbon dioxide, small, roundish colonies appear—*each* of which represents the astronomic progeny of a *single* bacterium. That is, each colony is a "pure" growth. Of course not all the colonies are gonococci, and to pinpoint those which are, a solution of p-aminodimethylaniline monohydrochloride is poured over the surface of the chocolate agar. If the gonococcus is indeed present *its* colonies within minutes turn pink, then purple. As further confirmation, the "positive colonies" are added to various sugar solutions for evidence of fermentation. The gonococcus and the gonococcus alone ferments glucose and glucose alone. In contrast *Neisseria meningitidis* ferments *both* glucose and maltose, and so on.

An ideal culture medium would be one conducive to the propagation of the gonococcus and the gonococcus alone—a "selective medium," to use the laboratory expression. And in 1966 J. D. Thayer and J. E. Martin succeeded in concocting such a medium from a rich assortment of nutrients plus three antibiotics—vancomycin, colistimethate, and nystatin. Ideally, these particular antibiotics prevent the multiplication of the usual contaminating inhabitants of the urogenital pathways but do not prevent the multiplication of *Neisseria gonorrhoeae*. Provided the technical personnel are thoroughly familiar with all the in's and out's of this new approach, the Thayer-Martin, or T-M, medium, as it is called, certainly facilitates the laboratory diagnosis.

Another interesting development relates directly to the doctor's office, to the actual taking of the specimen. The idea is to get the specimen to the laboratory at the earliest possible hour lest the gonococci—if present—perish on the way and destroy the diagnosis. This has always been a problem, because the gonococcus, as we know, is such a frail, fussy microbe. Available now is a transport medium aptly called "Transgrow," a modified Thayer-Martin formula in screw-capped bottles having an atmosphere of 10 percent carbon dioxide (CO_2). The medium is inoculated by removing the screw cap and rolling a swab containing the specimen over the surface of the agar, making sure the mouth of the bottle is kept elevated to minimize the loss of CO_2. After transportation to a central laboratory the bottle is incubated at 95-96°F. for 24 hours. Negative bottles (no growth on the medium) are reincubated for an additional 24 hours. Gonococci should remain viable for 48 to 96 hours in transit, and this time may be appreciably extended by incubating the bottle at 95° to 96°F. prior to mailing. Indeed, a prior incubation time of 16 to 18 hours will produce a growth that will be ready for definitive examination *immediately* upon arrival at the laboratory. Thus, for the first time, a highly sensitive means of diagnosing gonorrhea in the asymptomatic female will be available for use by the physician in the rural or outlying areas who does not have ready access to a bacteriology laboratory.

And the revered gram stain itself may some day go the way of the dodo, for already a number of laboratories are employing the "fluorescent antibody technique" (FAT). Briefly, gonococcal antibody (produced by inoculating gonococci into animals and then harvesting the blood serum) is combined with fluorescein to produce a "tagged" antibody, just as in the FADF test for syphilis. Thus, when a solution of tagged antibody is poured over the smear in question and then gently rinsed away, gonococci—if present—will *glow* under the ultraviolet microscope. As explained earlier, this is because antibody only "attacks" and remains attached to the antigen (the gonococcus in this case) that provoked it. All other microbes will not glow.

The real diagnostic answer to gonorrhea, however, will almost have to be a good serologic test, because such a test is the only one that can spot telltale antibodies in the symptom-free purveyor of disease. Equally important, a serologic test can be used to screen specimens *anonymously* in the course of systematic and routine investigations. Up until rather recently the prospects were not promising in this laboratory approach, but now all of a sudden several such tests augur some kind of breakthrough. According to the Center for Disease Control three methods have emerged as the most feasible—a flocculation test (similar to the VDRL), a complement-fixation test, and an indirect fluorescent antibody test (a takeoff on the FTA-ABS test for syphilis). Studies currently are evaluating each of these in terms of sensitivity and specificity and field evaluations are now being carried out in several cities. . . . Soon we shall know.

11
Penicillin, Again

The 1924 edition of *The Household Physician* tells the reader to treat appendicitis with a big dose of magnesium citrate—a cathartic par excellence! And its advice on "clap" is equally arresting. ". . . . Warm baths, warm sweating drinks . . . . holding the penis in warm water . . . . applying leeches to the scrotum . . . . walking barefooted upon the cold floor. . . ." Medicamentwise, too, there is much imagination in this particular tome—potassa, tartar emetic, camphor, opium, hyoscyamus, copaiba, cubebs, not to mention an avalanche of polypharmic concoctions—*Prescriptions* "120," "207," "208," "272," and on and on. Copaiba and cubeb were especially revered, the former being by far and away the major V.D. remedy in Civil War medicine. As one Washington newspaper noted, "The prostitutes fasten onto every soldier who is at all susceptible and stick with the tenacity of leeches until they convey them to their haunts of iniquity. . . . *Quinine* may be the need of the Confederate army, but *copaiba* is certainly the necessity of ours." [italics mine]

Copaiba, a thick, yellowish-brown, spicy-smelling liquid with an ungodly taste (derived from the tree *Copaifera officinalis* of tropical America) *does* impart a modicum of antisepsis to the urine and probably did on occasion ameliorate a burning gonococcal urethra. And to a degree the same applies to cubeb, the pleasant tasting unripe fruit of the piperaceous Java plant, *Piper cubeba.* (The pepper of "salt and pepper" is the dried fruit of *Piper nigrum.*) Further, cubeb doubled as an all purpose remedy for respiratory complaints and at one time the cubeb cigarette, "cubebs," was a leading brand. According to *The Household Physician,* then, the clap patient of the Roaring Twenties could do little better than keeping the feet cool and the private parts warm while puffing away on cubeb.

Less facetiously, medicine did possess silver, and "silver injections" did effect "speedy" cures in the *initial* phases of the disease when the gonococci were confined to the urethra. The "injections" consisted of instilling solutions of silver nitrate and/or Argyrol (silver protein) directly into the urethra three or four times a day and holding it there ten minutes or so per instillation. Doctor James Mumford of the Massachusetts General Hospital had great faith in 20 percent Argyrol and in the 1911 edition of his *Practice of Surgery* we read, "Argyrol thus used (as 20 percent injections) will cut short many cases of gonorrhea, sometimes limiting the duration of the attack to *a week or ten days.*" [italics mine] About deeper involvements and complications and chronic chronic gonorrhea ("gleet") he was not very reassuring. "*When* is the patient cured?" asks Doctor Mumford. ". . . . *When,*" he quotes a Doctor Whitney, "there is no longer a discharge, *when* the shreds [in the urine] contain neither pus, gonococci, nor a large amount of epithelium [urethral lining]; and *when,* furthermore, after producing a discharge by silver nitrate, no organisms are present;

when, after alcohol or sexual excess, no discharge appears." [italics all mine]

Jumping now from copaiba and cubebs and Argyrol to penicillin, we encounter the disquieting medical news that over the past several years *Neisseria gonorrhoeae* has been developing resistance to the moldy panacea. In Vietnam penicillin fails to cure about 25 percent of the cases of gonorrhea and here at home similar failures are cropping up all over the country, very serious resistant problems having been reported in California. Some credit the difficulty to the immigration of exotic strains from Vietnam and elsewhere, but most authorities simply look upon the situation as microbial Darwinism occasioned by *inadequate* dosage. Put bluntly, if a shot of penicillin is not potent enough to destroy *all* gonococci the resistant survivors in time predominate. And this is what has probably happened in Vietnam where a *little* penicillin is available to the man in the street.

In the words of the United States Public Health Service, "The treatment of gonorrhea is in a state of uncertainty although penicillin still remains the drug of choice." The "official" regimen runs as follows: For uncomplicated gonorrhea in men 2.4 million units of aqueous procaine penicillin G is given in one intramuscular injection (in the buttock); for uncomplicated gonorrhea in women, the dose (of the same drug) is 4.8 million units—half in each buttock.[1] Retreatment is indicated whenever discharge persists for three or more days following initial therapy and consists of doubling the original dosage at a single visit or in divided doses on two successive days. The management of complications calls

1. Women need more penicillin because the urine (the drug's "portal of exit") does not bathe all infection sites.

for large amounts of short acting ("soluble") penicillin. And patients who are sexual contacts to early syphilis should be given full prophylactic therapy for that disease (2.4 million units of long acting benzathine penicillin G) plus the recommended schedule for gonorrhea. Lastly, the Public Health Service considers tetracycline the substitute of choice in the event of gonococcal resistance and for patients hypersensitive to penicillin. The initial oral dose is 1.5 grams followed by 0.5 gram every six hours for four days, for a total of 9 grams.

Tetracycline and other broad spectrum antibiotics have proved to be over 90 to 95 percent effective in the treatment of gonorrhea and many venereal disease clinics are using these agents instead of penicillin. Another tactic is the concomitant use of a drug called probenecid (Benemid), a mainstay in the treatment of chronic gouty arthritis. On the one hand probenecid acts on the kidney to step up the excretion of uric acid (hence its value in gout) and on the other it *inhibits* the excretion of penicillin, thereby *raising and prolonging* the blood levels twofold to fourfold over conventional forms of administration. Probenecid also boosts the blood levels of related antibiotics, the U. S. Naval Preventive Medicine Unit 6 at Pearl Harbor reporting spectacular results using a *single oral dose* (3.5 grams) of ampicillin (Polycillin). *Without* probenecid, ampicillin was 71 percent successful. *With* probenecid, ampicillin was 96 percent successful!

Drug resistance, however, is by no means confined to penicillin. Most microbes in time develop some degree of resistance to just about any antibiotic, the towering exception being *Treponema pallidum*. A recent study in Toronto, Canada, for instance, showed 11 percent of the gonococci sampled to have developed resistance to tetracycline. Judging by past experience, it now seems advisable to isolate the infecting organism in every case of the disease and to determine in the laboratory its sensitivity not only to penicillin but also to the other antibiotics. Theoretically, all the antibiotics *now* in use will eventually prove worthless against gonorrhea, meaning that the chemist must always be at least one drug ahead of the game. So far he has been successful.

12
Preventives

For all intents and purposes the body possesses no defense against the gonococcus, notwithstanding the presence of antibody in the bloodstream of infected persons. What's more, gonorrhea can strike again and again and a new acute attack can actually superimpose itself on an old smoldering involvement. This poor immunologic showing plus the pathogen's silent omnipresence clearly means everlasting trouble. "Healthy" purveyors of *Neisseria gonorrhoeae* abound among females. Alas, even negative urogenital specimens do not *absolutely* rule out gonorrhea, for in chronic, deep-seated infections gonococci are sometimes here—"at the surface"—today and gone tomorrow. Lastly, we have no vaccine.

Thus, the control of gonorrhea, as of syphilis, centers on early diagnosis and speedy casefinding. Above all, routine testing should be implemented at every opportunity. For example, cultures for gonorrhea should be routine when women have pelvic examinations for other reasons. Of 164,000 women screened routinely in a wide variety of clinics during 1970, one in ten were found to be infected by the gonococcus!

Untreated gonorrhea is communicable for months and

often, especially in women, for years. On good authority and for the sake of precious time all contacts are considered "infected" and given penicillin (or tetracycline) at the earliest possible hour. According to the United States Public Health Service the prophylactic dose should be the same as the therapeutic dose, that is, 2.4 million units (of aqueous procaine penicillin G) for men, and 4.8 million units for women. Given during the incubation period, this invariably prevents gonorrhea. Indeed, if taken within three or four hours after exposure a *single tablet* of penicillin (25,000 units) *may* prevent gonorrhea![1]

The most dramatic development in the control and prevention of gonorrhea relates to gonorrheal conjunctivitis in the newborn or, *gonococcic ophthalmia neonatorum,* to use the sonorous medical Latin. At one time a leading cause of blindness throughout the world, it is today an uncommon occurrence in all enlightened countries and states calling for—*by law*—the "Credé treatment." Named after its creator, the German gynecologist Karl Sigmund Franz Credé (1819–1892), the original procedure called for placing one drop of 2 percent silver nitrate into each eye at *the time of delivery.* The modern version calls for one or two drops of 1 percent silver nitrate followed in a minute or two by enough warm saline (0.9 percent salt solution) to rinse it way. Silver nitrate, or "lunar caustic," to use the alchemistical designation, kills microbes on contact and to this day remains unexcelled for this purpose. But it is irritating (hence the saline wash) and has upon rare occasion caused eye injury. Also, accidents have occurred through errors (10

1. In the instance of *susceptible* strains, that is.

percent! instead of 1 percent, for instance). Consequently, most states allow the use of substitutes. The consensus though clearly favors the mystical, magical, lunar caustic.

Nonetheless, silver nitrate is by no means an *absolute* preventive against gonorrheal ophthalmia neonatorum, many investigators holding the revered chemical to be only partially effective. Recently, the Jules Stein Eye Institute (U.C.L.A. School of Medicine) reported the infection in two babies who had received the required silver nitrate drops at birth. Happily, both responded to a double barrel attack of penicillin intramuscularly and tetracycline topically.

In matters of personal prophylaxis the 1924 *Household Physician* renders reasonably sound advice, up to a point anyway. "The first requisite for prevention," we read, "is cleanliness. Before the act, the parts should be carefully examined to see if there be any breaks in the skin. The least breach in the covering of penis greatly promotes contagion. [Before the act] apply a solution of alum, tannin, or decoction of oak-bark and after act use acids or alkalies–vinegar and water is excellent . . . . Ricord (the famous French venereologist) uses wine with much success."

In point of fact just about any chemical agent kills gonococci and vinegar and wine are probably as good as any, although the experts favor soap and water. Standard procedure at the well-run house of prostitution, legal and otherwise, entails a good soap and water washing "of the parts" before and after–*plus condom.* How foolproof this really is remains anybody's guess. It sounds good and probably is good but we must never lose sight of what we might very properly dub the "all or none law." To wit, unless you kill *all* gonococci the gesture is conceivably no better than not killing any gonococci. One spirochete can cause syphilis. . . . One gonococcus can cause gonorrhea!

"LESSER" INVOLVEMENTS

13
Chancroid

The chancre, or primary sore, of syphilis fame is hard and painless and generally and surprisingly well recognized for what it is. In the old days even the laity in the more rough and tumble areas might acquire sufficient expertise to spot a chancre—a hard, syphilitic chancre—on sight. Accordingly chancres which were soft and painful came under increasing suspicion as being "something else." Indeed, the labels *soft chancre* and *chancroid* came into use and before long a new venereal disease was born. In 1889 the Italian dermatologist Augosto Ducrey added the vital touch by demonstrating the presence of tiny rod-shaped bacteria in the purulent discharge from such lesions and, what is more, proved their ability to incite chancroid when inoculated into the skin of the forearm. And in the very same year three French investigators, Doctors Besançon, Griffon, and Le Sourd, succeeded in culturing this new organism artificially.

Over the years Doctor Ducrey's pet pathogen received a great deal of laboratory scrutiny and today is officially relegated to a genus of bacteria aptly named *Hemophilus* —Greek, for "blood loving." That is, this tribe of bacteria

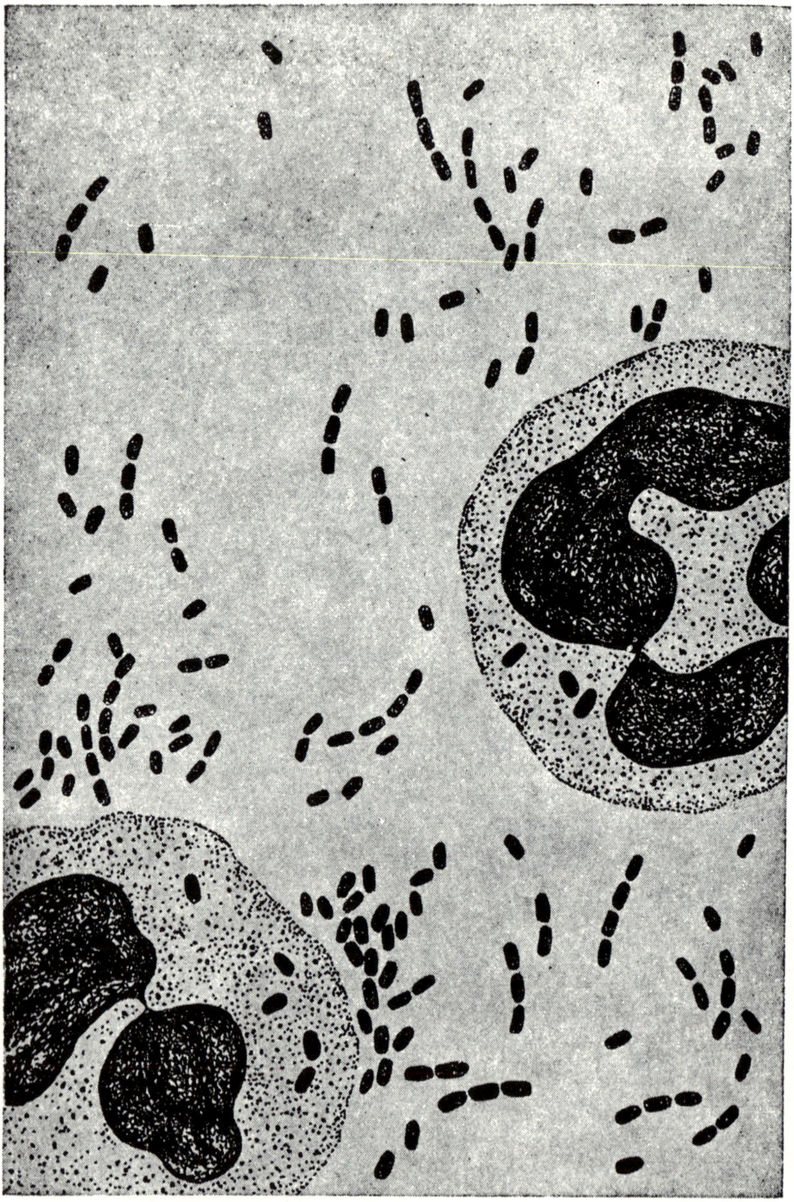

Hemophilus ducreyi in pus, showing dozens of the bacilli and two leukocytes (expanded 3,000x).

needs blood in order to grow. They are fastidious in other respects, too. For instance, although they need oxygen, the amount in the air (20 percent) is too much for them and has to be reduced. A number of "hemophili" are of medical concern. *Hemophilus influenzae* causes a type of meningitis; *Hemophilus aegyptius* causes a highly contagious conjunctivitis known as pink-eye; *Hemophilus duplex* causes blepharoconjunctivitis, a serious eye infection; and *Hemophilus ducreyi* causes, not surprisingly, chancroid, or soft chancre.

Chancroid occurs throughout the world and is especially common in tropical areas, overcrowded cities, and seaports. In the United States it has assumed an important V.D. role in the South, and the *reported* incidence for the country as a whole stood at 1,189 cases for 1970 (0.6 per 100,000 population). The disease is unique to man, although experimental animals, namely rabbits and monkeys, can be infected. Both man and animals develop hypersensitivity to the organism in the wake of an attack but fail to develop immunity against reinfection. Thus, chancroid, like gonorrhea, can strike again and again.

Three to five days (the *usual* interval) following sexual contact with an infected person a fiery pimple appears on the genitals or surrounding skin. Shortly thereafter this becomes pussy and necrotic and by a week's time develops into a soft, swollen, painful ulcer. There is plenty of infective ooze and this often sets off other chancroids via "autoinoculation." In *untreated* cases the rodlike invader makes its way into the lymph vessels leading to the lymph nodes and there, in the nodes, causes mean looking abscesses. At this point the infection turns systemic and constitutional and the patient feels "sick all over." Advanced cases may show chancroids elsewhere—the mouth and breasts appearing to be preferred sites.

According to some workers adequate evidence for the diagnosis of chancroid is the finding of tiny, gram-negative, blood-loving bacilli (rod-shaped bacteria) together with characteristic lesions and appropriate patient history. Additionally, others demand *positive* skin tests. In the "hypersensitive test" heat-killed *Hemophilus ducreyi* bacilli are injected into the skin and the injection site inspected at the end of 24 hours for the presence of a reaction. Those with chancroid become hypersensitive to the pathogen and display a reaction (positive test); all other persons ideally give no such reaction (negative test). In the autoinoculation test *chancroid* lesion fluid incites a chancroid when rubbed into scarified skin of the forearm.

A number of drugs inhibit and destroy *Hemophilus ducreyi* and rid the body of the disease, but just about all authorities cite the sulfonamides ("sulfas") as the drugs of choice. Control revolves around casefinding and intensive treatment of all contacts. For personal prophylaxis the condom is severely limited because the lesion or lesions are by no means confined to the penis. Plenty of soap and water "before and after," is certainly useful.

14
Granuloma Inguinale

Not uncommonly a hard chancre passes for a soft chancre and vice versa. Further, hard and soft chancres confuse and confound a venereal disease called *granuloma inguinale*, formerly known as "Donovania granulomatis" in honor of the Irish physician Charles Donovan. In smears and biopsy material taken from lesions suspected of being neither those of syphilis nor chancroid, Donovan discovered small, plump, rod-shaped bacteria which the laboratories throughout the world were soon to call "Donovan bodies." Only just recently did scientific sophistication rename the pathogen *Calymmatobacterium granulomatis.*

Granuloma inguinale is a chronic ulcerative disease transmitted through coitus and other forms of close body contact. Common in tropical areas and among the poverty stricken, the incidence in the United States dropped from 2,403 cases in 1947 to an all time low of 144 in 1965. The *reported* cases for 1968, 1969, and 1970 were 174, 126, and 168, respectively. The initial lesion, a swelling, appears at the pathogen's portal of entry on the genitals or often in the groin and anal area. Daughter lesions may then appear and with the passing of time rupture,

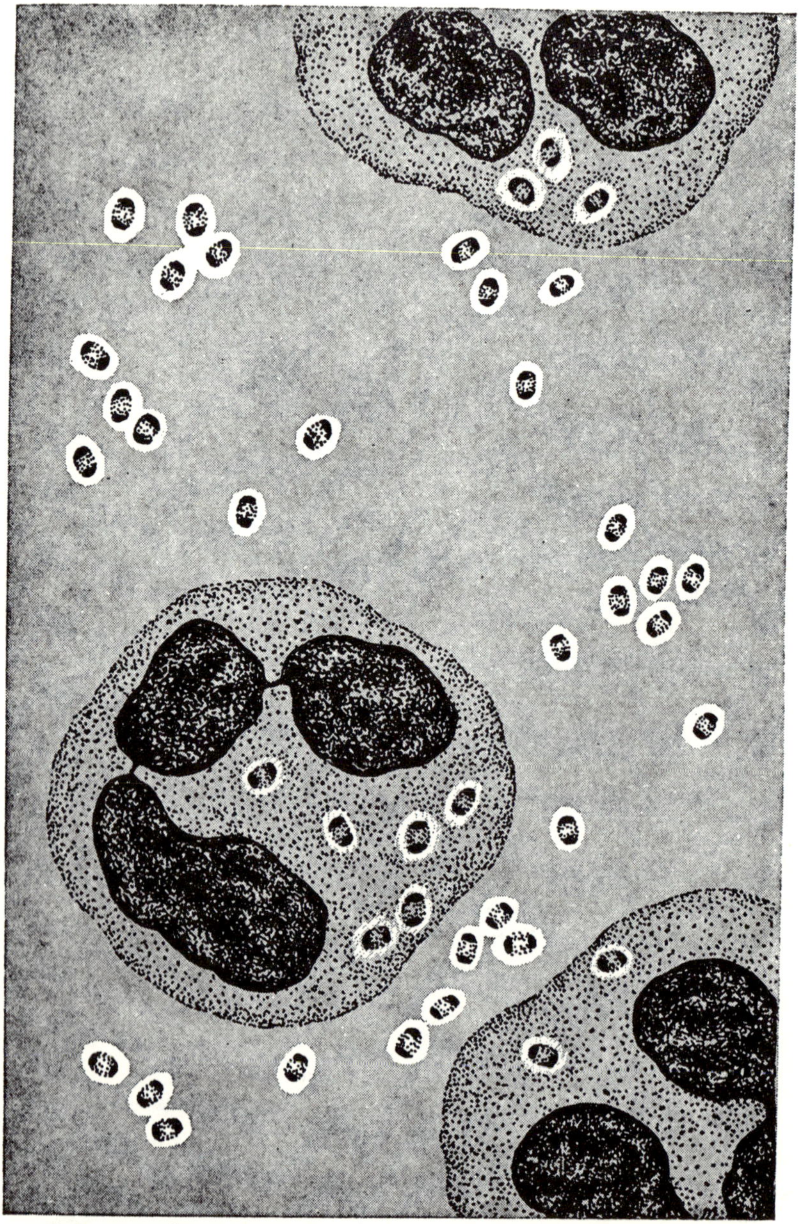

Calymmatobacterium granulomatis in pus. Note halo (capsule) surrounding organism and the three leukocytes ("pus cells"). Expanded 6,000x.

ulcerate, spread and coalesce, the destructive fetid process eventually involving the skin of the genitals, groin, buttocks, and lower abdomen. Sometimes there are systemic ramifications with arthritis and bone infection.

A diagnosis can be established only by demonstrating the presence of *Calymmatobacterium granulomatis* through the use of the appropriate microbiologic techniques. In the classic procedure, the one pioneered by Donovan, "lesion smears" are stained by the Wright method and then examined for small stocky dark blue bacilli ("rods") surrounded by a pinkish halo, or capsule, to use the laboratory word. And very typically these bacilli are crowded together within monocytes, the large white blood cells always present in this kind of ulcer. Stained according to the Gram method, the organism proves to be gram negative. Cultural characteristics are also critical and are absolutely essential when the direct smear or biopsy material is anything but enlightening. For this purpose the embryonated (fertile) egg is used plus an assortment of complex artificial media.

Granuloma inguinale yields to a number of antibotics, tetracycline and streptomycin generally heading the list in most tests. One schedule calls for 2 grams of tetracycline by mouth daily for two weeks or longer, depending upon the healing process. With respect to prevention and control, the approach parallels what's been said before—casefinding and immediate and intensive treatment of all contacts. Individual prophylaxis once again centers on a good washing of the genitals and surrounding area with plenty of soap and water.

15
LGV

The classification of living things (the science of taxonomy) is a vexatious job, particularly when dealing with the microbial world where things look and behave so much alike. Often a given species is classified as such and such mainly for convenience, which is certainly the case in the instance of *Treponema pallidum.* Although officially pigeonholed with the bacteria (as are all spirochetes) its pronounced motility is clearly remindful of one-celled animals, or protozoa. Bacteria are one-celled *plants*! Stated another way, for a number of technical reasons spirochetes are closer to bacteria than they are to protozoa—ergo, they are "bacteria."

But perhaps the best way to underscore this business of taxonomic musical chairs concerns the venereal disease at hand—lymphogranuloma venereum (or LGV). For a good thirty years the etiologic pathogen was considered a virus and then suddenly (*c.* 1960) the taxonomists relegated it to the rickettsiae. No one pretends to know where viruses belong in the scheme of things—indeed, even if they are "alive" or not—and as for the rickettsiae they occupy the twilight zone between viruses and bacteria. And now lo and behold the causative organism

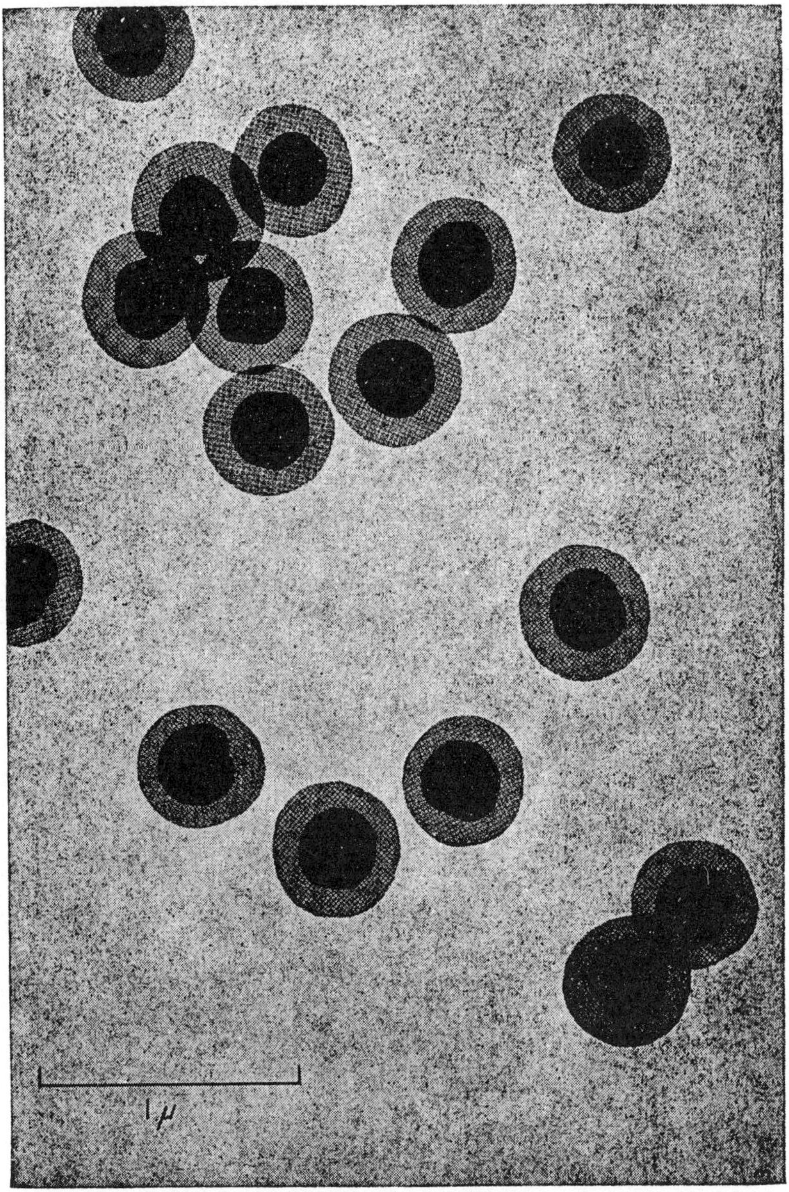

Bedsonia lymphogranulomatis as it appears under the electron microscope. The "line scale" at the bottom is one micron (μ), which is equal to 1/25,000 inch.

has been transferred again, this time to the *Bedsoniae,* another twilight family of pathogens situated somewhere between the rickettsiae and bacteria. By way of a name, the LGV bug was first called a "virus," then exotic *Miyagawanella lymphogranulomatis* (in its rickettsial days) and now *Bedsonia lymphogranulomatis.*

LGV was first described as a clinical entity in 1913 by three French physicians, Jean Durand, Joseph Nicolas, and M. Favre, and the medical dictionary still carries the entry "Durand-Nicolas-Favre Disease." Other extant synonyms are, among others, lymphogranuloma inguinale, tropical bubo, and climatic bubo. The disease's "viral" etiology was recognized in the 1930s, and within recent years *Bedsonia lymphogranulomatis* has been cultured successfully in the embryonated hen's egg and photographed under the electron microscope. LGV occurs throughout the world, but is most common in tropical regions and poverty stricken cities and towns. In this country it is endemic in the southern regions bordering the Gulf of Mexico and during World War II the incidence among Blacks in certain areas ran as high as 40 percent of those examined. In 1944 LGV hit an all time high of 2,858 cases and since that time has dropped in a seesaw fashion. For fiscal year 1970, 587 cases were reported to the United States Public Health Service.

Following sexual exposure *Bedsonia lymphogranulomatis* appears throughout the fluids and tissues and the primary lesion is noted in a couple of weeks or so. In the male the lesion usually takes the form of a blister on the foreskin or head of the penis, and in the female blisters pop up on the vulva, vaginal wall, and cervix. And in both sexes such lesions may attack the urethra and anal area. Shortly, these blisters break down, ulcerate, and then heal without scarring. Meanwhile, the pathogen has been up to considerable mischief in the regional lymph nodes, which in a matter of days become enlarged and terribly painful. Often these suppurate, break through the skin and discharge a foul pus. Sometimes discharge goes on for weeks and months. And systemically all is not well. Fever, general aches and pains, and arthritis are common. Occasionally, there may be conjunctivitis, and rarely meningitis and pericarditis (inflammation of the sac enclosing the heart). Eventually everything clears up, or appears to anyway, and for some victims their bout with LGV is over for good. In others *Bedsonia lymphogranulomatis* is merely taking an extended rest period and strikes again years later, the return involvement taking the form of chronic ulcerative lesions about the genitalia and rectum. In the female there may be rectal strictures, severe enough in some cases to require surgery. The lymphatic vessels are usually obstructed, the watery tissue fluid they normally drain away to the blood accumulating to cause grotesque swellings (elephantiasis) of the vulva, scrotum, and penis. And atop these tardy repercussions the patient may develop an overwhelming anemia and start to waste away. He could die!

LGV looks very much like chancroid and a number of other diseases marked by the formation of buboes in the groin area. Nonetheless a diagnosis can usually be made without difficulty via serology and the Frei skin test. The chief serologic test is based on the presence of complement-fixation antibodies in the blood of infected persons. The Frei skin test, named for its originator, the German dermatologist Wilhelm Frei, is based upon the development of hypersensitivity of infected persons to a "test antigen" (marketed as *Lygranum*) prepared from the organism *Bedsonia lymphogranulomatis* cultivated in the chick embryo. In practically every patient a reaction develops in a week or two at the site of the injection (usually the skin of the forearm). However, the result must always be viewed with caution. A positive test often persists from previously *cured* infections, and certain "chemically related" infections, parrot fever (psittacosis), for instance, give a positive test. The lesions themselves are diagnostic and the seasoned pathologist can spot LGV from the way biopsy material appears under the microscope.

Treatment entails the use of sulfonamides and tetracycline, both of which generally effect dramatic results. According to one schedule, sulfisoxazole (Gantrisin) is given at a dose of 4 grams daily over a three-week period. Additionally, buboes may have to be drained and surgery may be needed to correct strictures and the derangements of elephantiasis. No vaccine is available, so control and prevention at the public health level are a matter of case-finding and immediate treatment of contacts. At the individual level it is a matter of lots of soap and water in the wake of sexual intercourse.

16
Listeriosis

Back in 1926 a strange malady turned up in rabbits and guinea pigs characterized chiefly by a tremendous increase in *monocytes* (white blood cells with a large bean-shaped nucleus). Shortly thereafter the causative organism was isolated—a gram positive rod-shaped bacterium sporting a whiplike propeller (flagellum). In 1929 the pathogen turned up in a human being suffering from meningitis. Originally christened *Bacterium monocytogenes* the microbe is known officially today as *Listeria monocytogenes* (after Lord Lister, the "father of antiseptic surgery"). The disease itself is called listeriosis.

Over the years listeriosis has picked up more and more coverage in both medical and bacteriological texts. The disease is now known to be anything but uncommon and occurs throughout the animal world, the epidemiologic reservoir. Humans usually get the infection from animals via handling and contaminated food products—hence the higher prevalence in rural areas—but can and do pass it on to each other via close body contact. The pathogen frequents the private parts and venereal listeriosis is certainly much more common than even the doctors realize. Actually, the disease's natural history is

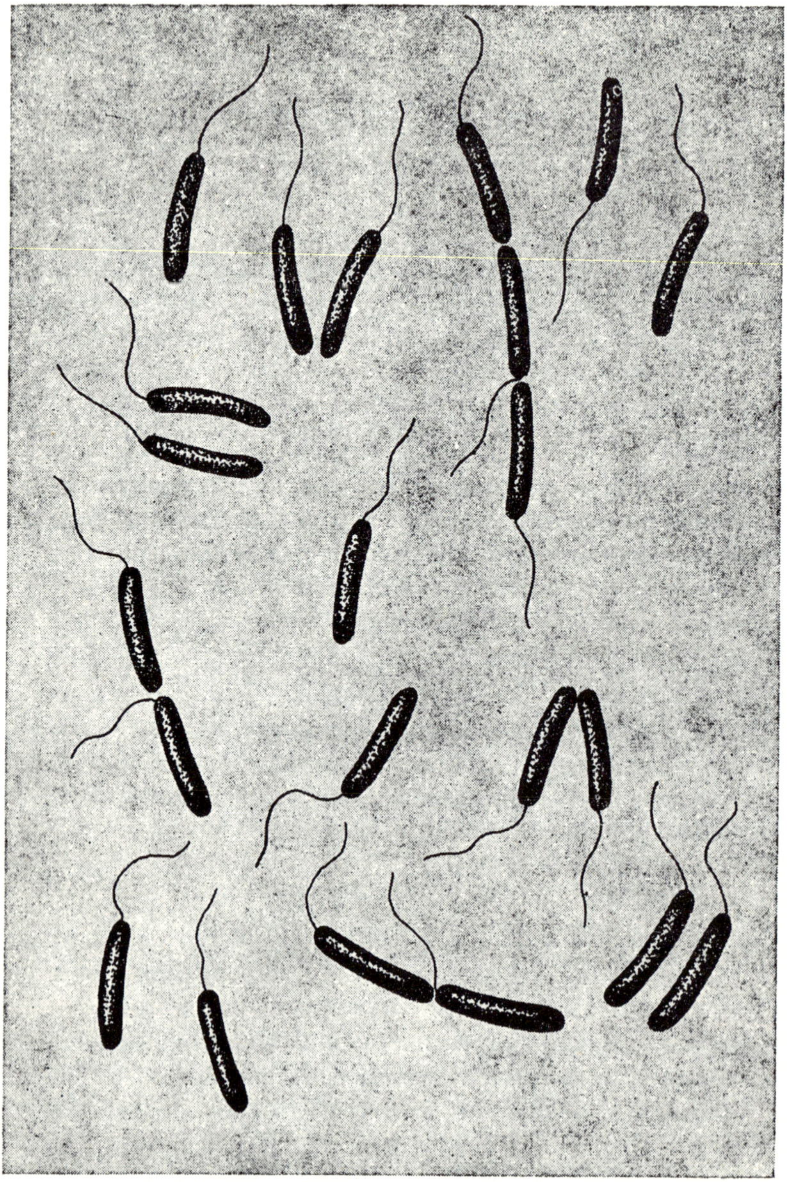

Listeria monocytogenes (expanded 6,000x).

protean and capricious and extraordinarily confusing. Depending on the circumstances it can pass for pneumonia, influenza, infectious mononucleosis, and encephalitis, to mention a few. In the main, though, listeriosis takes the form of a severe meningitis with all its horrors—nausea, vomiting, stupor, convulsions, and sometimes death.

Interestingly, *Listeria monocytogenes* encounters considerable resistance in healthy tissue and often fails to cause trouble even when habitually present, say in the vagina or under the foreskin. Indeed, this situation, known to microbiology as commensalism, is parasitism at its highest, because when you stop to think about it why should any parasite want to do away with host and home. But as just suggested the host may get sick from other causes—from another pathogen!—the ensuing unhealthy tissue then falling prey to the perennial guest. And most important the infected pregnant woman may infect the fetus and cause abortion and stillbirth. Of those who survive the prenatal period some emerge with multiple abscesses and others with meningitis.

The diagnosis is made by demonstrating gram positive rod-shaped microbes in the culturings of suitable specimens, and the use of special tests, such as the ability of *Listeria monocytogenes* to cause a characteristic conjunctivitis when instilled into a rabbit's eye. Therapeutically, tetracycline produces good results, and prophylactically the best we can do is to be on guard against the unexpected and inexplicable.

17

Trichomonas Vaginitis

Quite contrary to what many seem to believe, microorganisms are basically our friends. Without them the planet Earth would soon grind to a halt. And nowhere is this ecological state of affairs brought closer to home than among the microbial populations of the human body. All kinds and sorts of bacteria and fungi compose the "normal flora" of the skin and all kinds and sorts of bacteria and fungi and protozoa compose the "normal flora" of the gastrointestinal and urogenital tracts. The penis and vagina are veritable microbial gardens. To be sure the vast majority of resident species are the "good guys," always keeping in check the "bad guys." That is why we say the *normal* flora.

Of particular importance is a tribe of vaginal bacteria called lactobacilli, the waste products of which make the vaginal secretions acidic—acidic enough to inhibit and keep *in check* a one-celled animal malefactor by the name of *Trichomonas vaginalis*. Discovered in 1837 by the French physician Alfred Donné, *Trichomonas vaginalis* is believed to inhabit the vagina and male urethra of a good quarter of the population, causing trouble in the female—it almost never bothers the male—when something comes along to upset the ecologic balance normally enforced by the lactobacilli. Big doses of antibotics can do it by killing off the lactobacilli. Overdouching can do it by rinsing away both lactobacilli and their acid products. The menopause can do it with its changed "normal flora" and fewer lactobacilli. The symptomless, healthy male can do it by ejaculating contaminated semen. Moreover, once the infection—known to medicine as trichomonas vagin*itis* and trichomoniasis—is established, sexual intercourse keeps it going. In the view of many authorities "man and wife" trichomoniasis is our most common venereal disease!

Untreated trichomoniasis can be a real problem. The vagina and vulva may itch beyond belief and a profuse, foamy, foul-smelling, yellowish discharge makes its way to the surface. The psychological ramifications can be considerable. Making the diagnosis is generally easy because the discharge teems with *Trichomonas vaginalis,* one of the goofiest looking creatures known to the art and science of microscopy. It is a good size pear-shaped protozoan (one-celled animal) sporting four whiplike projections, or flagella, at the head and a fifth flagellum along the outer margin of a highly characteristic undulating membrane. These structures impart mobility and in so-called "wet mounts" the parasite can be seen clearly revolving and paddling and wobbling along its mischievous ways.

Whereas once upon a time the treatment of trichomoniasis was long and drawn out and commonly unsuccessful, the cure rate today runs close to 100 percent, just about the epitome of chemotherapy. And in this instance the wonder drug is metronidazole, marketed by G. D. Searle and Co. under the imaginative brand name *Flagyl.*

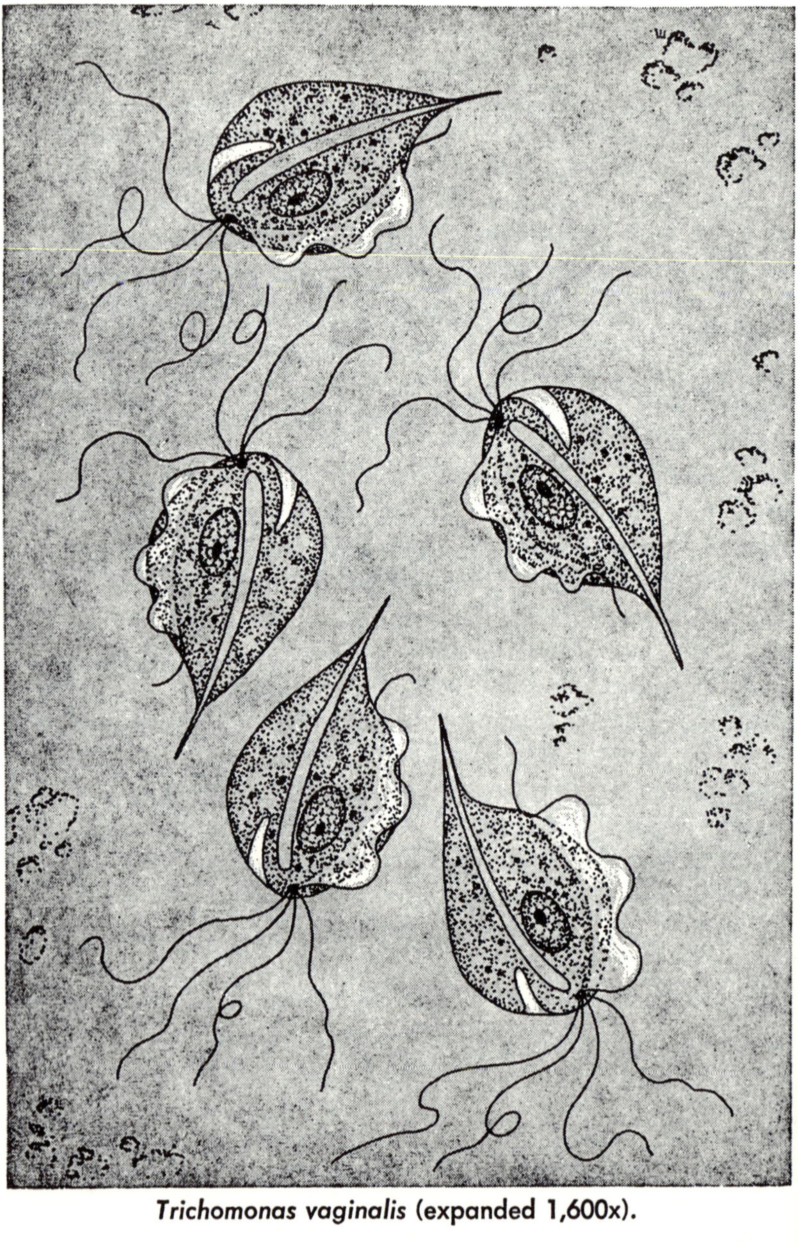

Trichomonas vaginalis (expanded 1,600x).

A trichomonacide par excellence, Flagyl acts systemically to eradicate trichomonads sequestered in the inner recesses of the urogenital tract of both sexes. The recommended schedule in the female is one 250 milligram tablet orally three times daily for ten days. In the few cases where repeat courses of the drug are called for, it is recommended that an interval of four to six weeks elapse between courses and that a white blood cell count be made before, during, and after treatment. In very stubborn cases 500 milligram vaginal inserts are used in addition to the tablet. In the male Flagyl is prescribed only in the presence of trichomonads—one 250 milligram tablet two times daily for ten days. When prescribed for the male in conjunction with the treatment of his consort the medication to be effective must be taken by *both* partners over the *same* ten day period.

Trichomonas vaginalis is by no means the only species of the genus. Harmless brothers and sisters abound and two are well known to human biology. One, *Trichomonas hominis,* inhabits the intestine and another, *Trichomonas buccalis,* frequents the mouth. Thus, relative to the genus *Trichomonas,* the sexual act affords interesting microbial possibilities.

18
Crab Lice

Lice are wingless insect vampires inhabiting the skin and hair of mammals. They are blind as a bat, have flattened bodies, and possess an extensible mouth well adapted for piercing skin and sucking blood. Two species are of medical concern—*Pediculus humanus* and *Phthirus pubis. Pediculus humanus* comes in two biologic *varieties* (abbreviated var.). One, *Pediculus humanus* var. *capitis,* infests the head ("head louse"), and the other, *Pediculus humanus* var. *corporis* infests clothing and the body at large, particularly the hair of the chest. And *Phthirus pubis* (the "crab louse"), a final parasitic star in our "V.D. Story," infests, as its name indicates, the pubic area.

Crab lice may indeed be blind but the warmth and smell of blood and hair bring them on the run to just the right spot, to their "ecological niche" as it were. Infested clothing and body contact transfer the elegant vermin, and most especially the sexual act with its vigorous intermingling of pubic hairs. Once residence has been established and food and shelter assured, the male crab louse jumps the female crab louse and thrusts its chitinous pointed penis into the appropriate orifice to effect fertilization. At the proper time the pregnant female deposits her fertile sticky eggs, or nits, on the hair where in a matter of days they evolve into nymphs, or what appear to be Peter Pan adults. Subsequent changes occur and in about a month's time sexually mature lice are at hand to perpetuate and expand the species. In severe infestations the population explosion extends to the armpits, chest hairs, and even eyebrows and eye lashes. The bites and epidermal response to parasite saliva and excreta provoke intense itching and scratching, the upshot being a roseate dermatitis embellished with crusts and matted hair.

The hapless host can easily identify and diagnose the situation. The nits show up as pubic dandruff and the six-legged critters, which run a sixteenth of an inch or so, can be hunted down with a fine-toothed comb. Those on the eyelashes may well appear as monsters on the horizon. The lay language labels are "lice" among the upper class and "crabs" among the lower. The general practitioner politely calls it pediculosis and the dermatologist, phthiriasis.

One can well appreciate the pharmaceutic lengths man has gone to destroy *Phthirus pubis*. Larkspur, carbolic acid, sulfur, chewing tobacco, kerosene, camphor, vinegar, and mercury merely give an idea. A revered remedy for years was "blue ointment," a concoction of finely divided mercury metal dispersed in a base of petroleum jelly. During both world wars a favorite refrain at sick call was "Get Out the Old Blue Ointment to the Crab's Disappointment." But as in all such matters it remained for the organic chemist to conquer lice and this he did

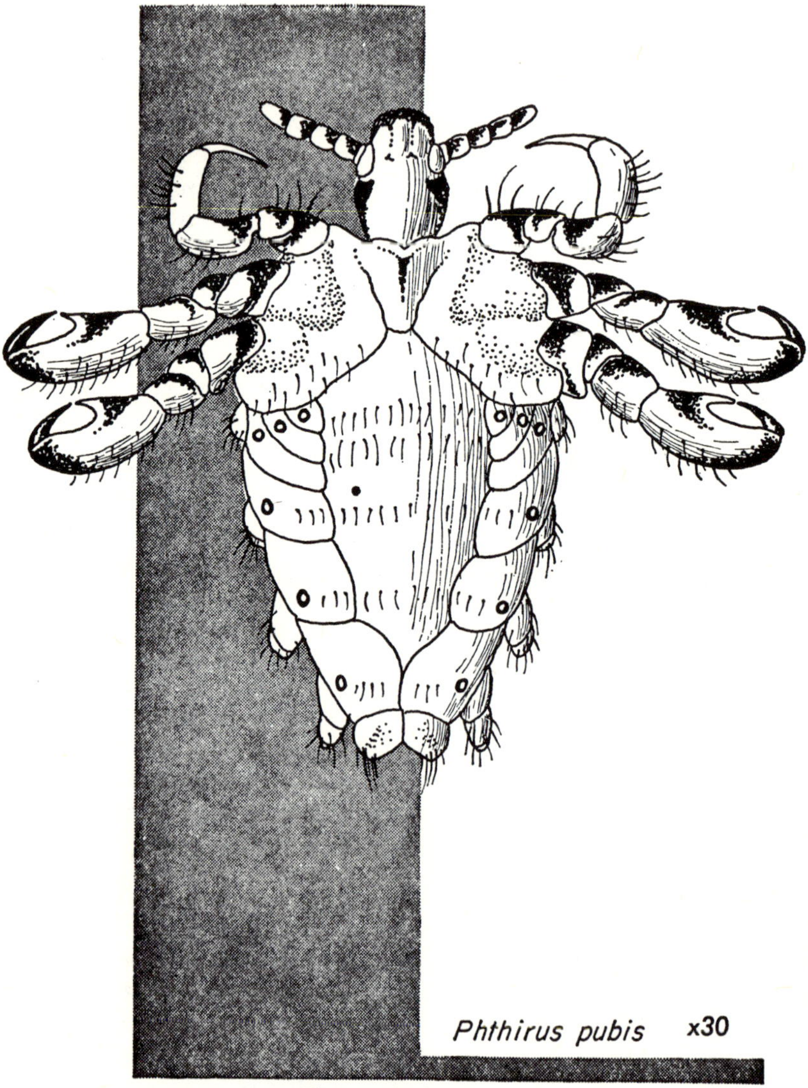

The crab louse.

with the magic molecule gamma benzene hexachloride. Marketed under the name "Kwell" at a 1 percent concentration, a single application of the cream or lotion is frequently all that is needed to wipe out the parasite. Certainly, it is a happy ending to at least one V.D. Story.

19

Cancer

What you might call our taxonomic tally up to the present and last chapter amounts to this: Bacteria cause syphilis, gonorrhea, chancroid, granuloma inguinale, and listeriosis; a bedsonian causes lymphogranuloma venereum; a protozoan causes trichomonas vaginitis; and an insect causes pediculosis. Now we come to the one and only V.D. *viral* pathogen—the "cold sore virus." But before we talk about the cold sore virus, let us first take a brief look at the world of the viruses.

As pointed out before, no one knows where viruses *belong* in the scheme of living things. With no play on words they straddle the fence between life and death. But this is not to say that we know little *about* viruses, for actually we know more about viruses than any other group of microbes. And the gist of what we know is this: A virus particle—or virion, as it is called—is composed of a huge molecule of genetic substance surrounded by a protein coat called a capsid. When a virion invades a living cell the genetic substance takes over. In some instances, the "injected" genetic substance orders the *cell's* genetic apparatus to make more virions, which upon release from the destroyed host proceed to infect neighboring cells in a chain reaction manner. In other instances, the two genetic systems "fuse" to produce a wayward cell. The clinical upshot is disease—either infection or cancer! Although the etiologic relationship of viruses to cancer in animals is well established, the situation in man still remains circumstantial. All evidence points to the virus as a key causal factor, but as of this writing no one has dotted all the i's and crossed all the t's at the laboratory level.

Relative to *each other* viruses are classified with what you might call arithmetic precision, certainly with a precision not obtaining in any other taxonomic area. Three major points are considered—the nature of the genetic substance, the size of the virion, and the design of the capsid. In regard to genetic substance a virus possesses *either* deoxyribonucleic acid (DNA) or ribonucleic acid (RNA)—*never* both. In regard to size, virions range from some 10 millimicrons to some 200 millimicrons. (It takes 25 million millimicrons to span an inch!) And in regard to the capsid, the latter is divided into distinct individual subunits called capsomeres—a given virus having a set number.

Screened in the framework of the foregoing criteria, animal viruses compose thirteen groups, one of which is our concern here—herpesvirus. Herpesviruses are "large" DNA virions (averaging some 110 millimicrons[1]) whose capsids are fashioned into exactly 162 capsomeres. Several "species" cause disease in man, notably the VZ virus and the herpes simplex virus. The first invasion of the body by the VZ virus causes chickenpox (varicella), whereas shingles (or herpes zoster) results from the activation of

1. This refers to the naked virion; "enveloped" virions, those surrounded by a limiting membrane, range from 180 to 250 millimicrons.

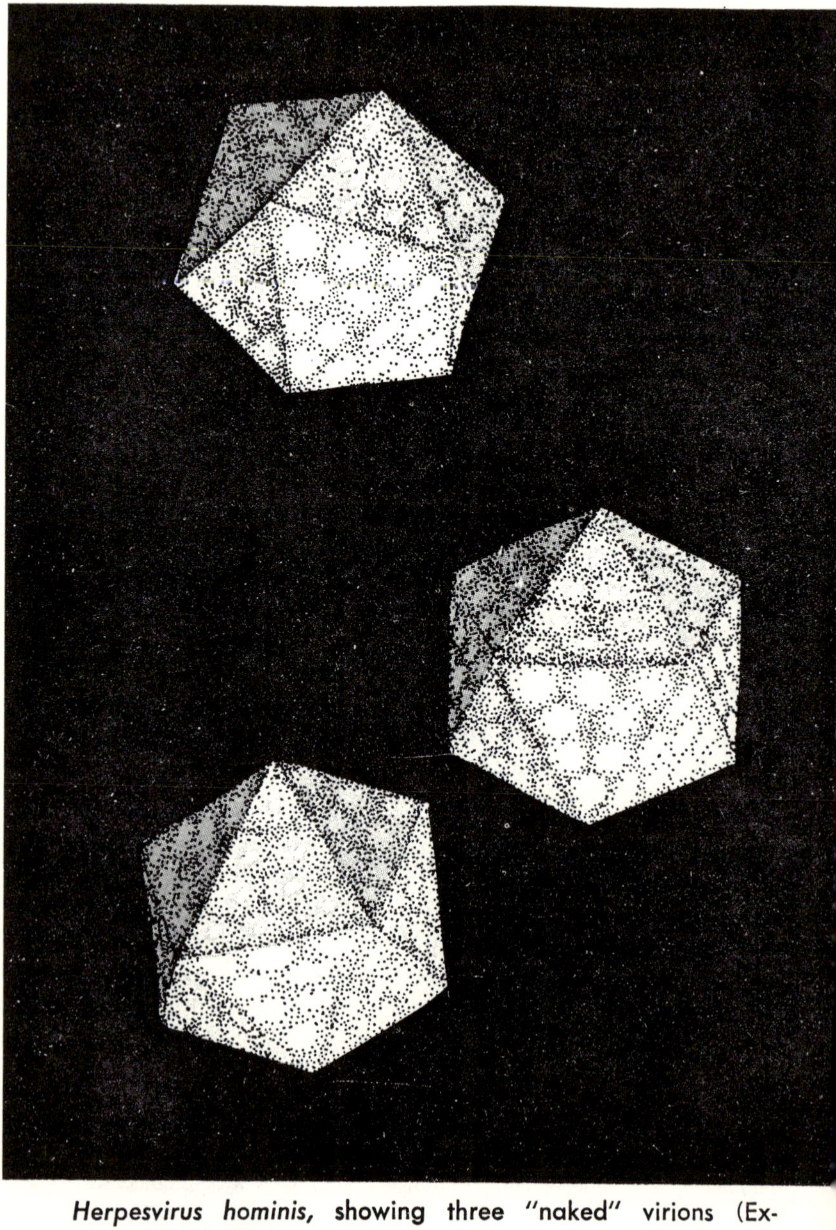

Herpesvirus hominis, showing three "naked" virions (Expanded 600,000x)

the latent virus. The herpes simplex virus (also called *Herpesvirus hominis* or HVH for short) causes herpes simplex, an acute infection marked by water blisters on the skin and mucous membranes—the classic lesion being the cold sore.

Herpes simplex of the genital mucosa has been recognized since time immemorial, but not until the past dozen years or so has it entered the venereal limelight. Now there is a mushrooming of reports and surveys attesting to the venereal transfer of HVH type 2. (HVH type 1 is almost exclusively associated with the mouth and the cold sore.) In one clearcut study seven out of eight female contacts of seven males with herpetic infections of the penis showed evidence of HVH type 2 genital infection. As for prevalence, several VD clinics report HVH type 2 is the most common cause of genital lesions in females and second only to primary syphilis as the cause of such lesions (blisters and ulcers) in men. And at one V.D. clinic teenagers have been found to account for about one half of the cases of genital herpetic infections. Also, HVH type 2 and upon occasion HVH type 1 cause "herpes simplex neonatorum," a usually fatal disease of the newborn marked by destructive lesions of the liver and brain. Presumably, the baby encounters the virus in the birth canal during delivery.

But the most startling herpetic news relates to the rapidly accumulating evidence that cancer of the cervix is caused by HVH type 2. According to highly authoritative sources three out of four women who have had genital herpes go on to develop this morbid condition. Further, the venereal implications are substantial and impressive. Uncircumcised male partners, multiple marriages, multiple sex partners, and early age of first coitus are all associated with an increased incidence. Indeed, cervical cancer is least common in virgins and most common in prostitutes. Accordingly, the socioeconomic findings are hardly surprising; namely, the prevalence of genital herpes is about one in 3,000 among the rich, compared to one in 250 among the poor. And at the test tube level we encounter the interesting matter of hormones. That is, since genital herpes is about as common in men as in women *perhaps* female hormones account for the relative commonness of cervical cancer in women and rarity of penile cancer in men. More particularly, perhaps female hormones lay the chemical groundwork for a successful attack by HVH type 2. Needless to say, "the pill" is under close scrutiny.

In light of these revelations and the seriousness of cervical cancer (the third most common cause of cancer deaths in women), the experts are recommending check-ups every six months among women with diagnosed genital herpes or who are found through routine "pap tests" to harbor HVH type 2. Moreover, the women and the doctors will have to pay more attention to the infection itself, especially since most cases of genital herpes are so minor as to escape notice.

And last and foremost, in the event HVH type 2 does prove to be the real culprit, a vaccine is conceivable—a vaccine to stimulate antibodies against herpes genitalis, indeed, a vaccine against "V.D. cancer."

Bibliography

Books

Alexander, H. E., Chancroid. *In* Beeson, P., and McDermott, W. (editors), *Cecil-Loeb; Textbook of Medicine,* 11th ed. Philadelphia: W. B. Saunders Co., 1963.

Anderson, W. A. D., and Scotti, T. M., *Synopsis of Pathology,* 7th ed. St. Louis: C. V. Mosby Co., 1968.

Bailey, R., and Scott, E. G., *Diagnostic Microbiology,* 2nd ed. St. Louis: C. V. Mosby Co., 1968.

Bauer, et al., *Bray's Clinical Laboratory Methods,* 7th ed. St. Louis: C. V. Mosby Co., 1968.

Beacham, D. W., and Beacham, W. D., *Synopsis of Gynecology,* 7th ed. St. Louis: C. V. Mosby Co., 1967.

Beeson and McDermott, *op. cit.*

Brooks, S. M., *A Programmed Introduction to Microbiology,* St. Louis: C. V. Mosby Co., 1968.

———. *Basic Facts of Medical Microbiology,* 2nd ed. Philadelphia: W. B. Saunders Co., 1962.

———. *Basic Facts of Pharmacology,* 2nd ed. Philadelphia: W. B. Saunders Co., 1963.

———. *Civil War Medicine.* Springfield, Ill.: Charles C Thomas, 1966.

———. *Integrated Basic Science,* 3rd ed. St. Louis: C. V. Mosby Co., 1970.

———. *The World of the Viruses.* South Brunswick, N. J. and New York: A. S. Barnes and Co., 1970.

Brown, H. W., Arthropods and Human Disease. *In* Beeson and McDermott, *op. cit.*

Brown, W. J., and Lucas, J. B., *Gonorrhea. In Practice of Medicine;* Loose-leaf Reference Service, by Frederick Tice, ed. by L. H. Sloan, New York: Harper and Row Publishers, 1967.

Burdon, K. L., and Williams, R., *Microbiology,* 6th ed. New York: Macmillan, 1968.

Burrows, W., *Textbook of Microbiology,* 19th ed. Philadelphia: W. B. Saunders Co., 1968.

Canizares, O., *Modern Diagnosis and Treatment of the Minor Venereal Diseases: The Management of Chancroid, Granuloma Inguinale, and Lymphogranuloma Venereum in General Practice.* Springfield, Ill.: Charles C Thomas, 1954.

Chandler, A. C., *Introduction to Parasitology,* 6th ed. New York: Wiley, 1940.

Clark, E. G., *Venereal Disease. In Preventive Medicine and Public Health* by Milton J. Rosenau, 9th ed. Edited by Philip E. Sartwell. New York: Appleton-Century Crofts, 1965.

Cluff, L. E., Listerosis. *In* Beeson and McDermott, *op. cit.*

Craig, C. F., and Faust, E. C., *Clinical Parasitology,* 2nd ed. Philadelphia: Lea and Febiger, 1940.

Culbertson, J. T., *Medical Parasitology.* New York: Columbia University Press, 1942.

Dennie, C. C., *A History of Syphilis.* Springfield, Ill.: Charles C Thomas, 1962.

Dodson, A. I., Jr., and Hill, J. E., *Synopsis of Genitouri-*

nary Disease, 7th ed. St. Louis: C. V. Mosby Co., 1962.

Dubos, R. J., and Hirsch, J. G. (eds.), *Bacterial and Mycotic Infections of Man,* 4th ed. Philadelphia: J. B. Lippincott, 1965.

Ewing, H. E. A., *A Manual of External Parasites.* Springfield, Ill.: Charles C Thomas, 1929.

Faust, E., and Russell, P. F., *Craig and Faust's Clinical Parasitology,* 7th ed. Philadelphia: Lea and Febiger, 1965.

Frankel, S. et al. (Editors), *Gradwohl's Clinical Laboratory Methods and Diagnosis,* 7th ed. St. Louis: C. V. Mosby Co., 1970.

Gardner, H. L., *Benign Diseases of the Vulva and Vagina.* St. Louis: C. V. Mosby Co., 1969.

Gebhardt, L. P., and Anderson, D., *Microbiology,* 3rd ed. St. Louis: C. V. Mosby Co., 1965.

Goodman, L. S., and Gilman, A., *The Pharmacological Basis of Therapeutics,* 3rd ed. New York: The Macmillan Co., 1965.

Hegner, R., and Taliaferro, W. H., *Human Protozoology.* New York: The Macmillan Co., 1929.

Hegner, R., et al., *Parasitology.* New York: Century, 1938.

Herms, W. B., *Medical Entomology,* 3rd ed. New York: The Macmillan Co., 1939.

Heyman, A., Lymphogranuloma venereum. *In* Beeson and McDermott, *op. cit.*

Horsfall, F. L., Jr., and Tamm, I. (Editors), *Viral and Rickettsial Infections of Man,* 4th ed. Philadelphia: J. B. Lippincott, 1965.

Household Physician, The (Many Editors), Buffalo: Brown-Flynn Publishing Co., 1924.

Hunter, G. W., Frye, W. W., and Swartzwelder, J. C.,

A Manual of Tropical Medicine, 4th ed. Philadelphia: W. B. Saunders Co., 1966.

Kirby, W. M., Gonococcal Disease. *In* Beeson and McDermott, *op. cit.*

Landon, J. F., and Sider, H. T., *Communicable Diseases.* Philadelphia: F. W. Davis, 1969.

McCormick, J. H., *Century Book of Health.* Springfield, Mass.: The King-Richardson Co., 1909.

McDermott, W., Granuloma Inguinale. *In* Beeson, P. and McDermott, *op. cit.*

———. Syphilis. *In ibid.*

Norins, L. C., and Wallace, A. L., Syphilis Serology Today. *In* Progress in Clinical Pathology. Vol. II, 1969 Grune and Stratton, Inc. New York.

Parran, T., *Shadows on the Land, Syphilis.* New York: Reynal and Hitchcock, 1937.

Peel, J., and Potts, M., *Textbook of Contraceptive Practice.* Cambridge: Cambridge University Press, 1969.

Pelczar, Jr., M. J., and Reid, R. D., *Microbiology,* 2nd ed. New York: McGraw-Hill Book Co., 1965.

Pusey, W. A., *History and Epidemiology of Syphilis.* Springfield, Ill.: Charles C Thomas, 1933.

Riley, W. A., and Johannsen, O. A., *Medical Entomology.* New York: McGraw-Hill Book Co., 1938.

Robbins, S. L., *Textbook of Pathology,* 2nd ed. Philadelphia: W. B. Saunders Co., 1962.

Smith, A. L., *Principles of Microbiology,* 5th ed. St. Louis: C. V. Mosby Co., 1965.

Sollmann, T., *A Manual of Pharmacology,* 8th ed. Philadelphia: W. B. Saunders Co., 1957.

Stanier, R. Y., Doudoroff, M., and Adelberg, E. A., *The Microbial World,* 2nd ed. Englewood Cliffs, N. J.: Prentice Hall, 1963.

Top, F. H., *Communicable and Infectious Diseases,* 6th ed. St. Louis: The C. V. Mosby Co., 1968.

Trussell, R. E., *Trichomonas Vaginalis and Trichomoniasis.* Springfield, Ill.: Charles C Thomas, 1947.

Wagner, R. R., Herpes Simplex. *In* Beeson and McDermott, *op. cit.*

Willcox, R. R., *Textbook of Venereal Diseases and Treponematoses,* 2nd ed. Springfield, Ill.: Charles C Thomas, 1964.

Wilson, M. E. and Mizer, H. E., *Microbiology in Nursing Practice.* New York: The Macmillan Co., 1969.

Journals

Alford, C. A., Jr., et al, "Gamma-M-Fluorescent Treponemal Antibody in the Diagnosis of Congenital Syphilis." *New England Journal of Medicine,* 280:1086, 1969.

Altman, R. D., "Recent Clinical Experience in the Management of Gonococcal Arthritis." *Journal of Florida Medical Association,* 56:318, 1969.

Amies, C. R., "Sensitivity of *Neisseria gonorrhoeae* to Penicillin and Other Antibiotics, Studies Carried Out in Toronto During the Period 1961 to 1968." *British Journal of Venereal Diseases,* 45:216, 1969.

Ashamalla, G., et al, "Recent Clinicolaboratory Observations in the Treatment of Acute Gonococcal Urethritis in Men." *Journal of the American Medical Association,* 195:1115, 1966.

Atwood, W. G., and Miller, J. L., "Fluorescent Treponemal Antibodies in Fractionated Syphilitic Sera. The Immunoglobulin Class." *Archives of Dermatology,* 100:763, 1969.

Beeler, M. F., et al, "Serologic Testing for Syphilis. Report From the Subcommittee on Serology of the Standards Committee of the College of American Pathologists." *American Journal of Clinical Pathology,* 52:300, 1969.

Beerman, H., et al, "Syphilis." *Archives of Internal Medicine,* 109:323, 1962.

Berggren, O., "Association of Carcinoma of the Uterine Cervix and *Trichomonas vaginalis* Infestations. Frequency of *Trichomonas vaginalis* in Preinvasive and Invasive Cervical Carcinoma." *American Journal of Obstetrics and Gynecology,* 105:166, 1969.

Boulton, H., "Significance of the 'Defaulter' in the Assessment of Efficiency of Treatment in Gonorrhoea." *British Journal of Venereal Diseases,* 45:40, 1969.

British Medical Research Council Report, "Resistance of Gonococci to Penicillin." *Lancet,* 2:226, 1961.

Brown, W. J., "Acquired Syphilis: Drugs and Blood Tests." *American Journal of Nursing,* 71:713, 1971.

———. "The Status of Gonorrhea in the United States of America and Current Problems in its Control." *Bulletin World Health Organization,* 24:386, 1961.

Brown, W. J. et al, "Experimental Syphilis in the Chimpanzee." *British Journal of Venereal Diseases,* 46:198, 1970.

Bunn, P. A., "Automicrobial Therapy in Patients Allergic to Penicillin." *New York Journal of Medicine,* 69:1859, 1969.

Catterall, R. D., "The Advance of Venereal Diseases." *Lancet,* 2:103, 1963.

Cave, V. G., "What's New in Venereal Disease." *Rhode Island Medical Journal,* 52:519, 1969.

Cave, V. G., et al, "Gonorrhea in the Obstetric and Gynecologic Clinic. Incidence in a Voluntary Hospital in an Urban Community." *Journal of the American Medical Association,* 210:309, 1969.

Cavenough, R. L., "The Serologic Syphilis Test Required for Marriage in Other States." *Maryland Medical Journal,* 18:33, 1969.

Center For Disease Control, State and Community Services Division. *VD Fact Sheet, 1970.* Basic Statistics On the Venereal Disease Problem in the United States, 27 ed. Atlanta.

Chacko, C. W., and Nair, G. M., "Sero-Diagnosis of Gonorrhea with a Microprecipitin Test Using a Lipopolysaccharide Antigen from *N. gonorrhoeae.*" *British Journal of Venereal Diseases,* 45:33, 1969.

Chandler, F. W., "A Technique for Detecting *Treponema pallidum* Through the Use of Membrane Filters and Immunofluorescence Staining." *British Journal of Venereal Diseases,* 45:305, 1969.

Cohen, D. S., et al, "Serum Antibody Response in Experimental Human Gonorrhoea." *British Journal of Venereal Diseases,* 45:325, 1969.

Cohen, P., et al, "Serologic Reactivity in Consecutive Patients Admitted to a General Hospital. A comparison of the FTA-ABS, VDRL and Automated Reagin Tests." *Archives of Internal Medicine,* 124:364, 1969.

"Condom: No Longer A Dirty Word." *Central Pharmaceutical Journal,* December 1970–January 1971.

Cowan, L., "Gonococcal Ulceration of the Tongue in the Gonococcal Dermatitis Syndrome." *British Journal of Venereal Diseases,* 45:228, 1969.

Creitz, J. R., et al, "Effectiveness of Transgrow Medium for *Neisseria meningitis.*" *Public Health Reports,* In Press.

Curtis, F. R., and Wilkinson, A. E., "A Comparison of the *In Vitro* Sensitivity of Gonococci to Penicillin with the Results of Treatment." *British Journal of Venereal Diseases,* 34:70, 1958.

Davis, C. M., and Collins, C., "Granuloma Inguinale: An Ultrastructural Study of *Calymmatobacterium granulomatis.*" *Journal of Investigative Dermatology,* 53:315, 1969.

Davis, C. M., "Granuloma Inguinale. A Clinical, Histological, and Ultrastructural Study." *Journal of the American Medical Association,* 211:632, 1970.

Deacon, W. E., "Fluorescent Antibody Methods for *Neisseria gonorrhoeae* Identification." *Bulletin of WHO,* 24:349, 1961.

Dewhurst, K., "The Neurosyphilitic Psychoses Today. A Survey of 91 Cases." *British Journal of Psychiatry,* 115:31, 1969.

Dienst, R. B., "New Preparations of Antigen for Intracutaneous Diagnosis of Chancroidal Infection." *American Journal of Syphilology,* 26:201, 1942.

Domescik, G., et al, "Use of a Single Oral Dose of Doxycycline Monohydrate for Treating Gonorrheal Urethritis in Men." *Public Health Reports,* 84:182, 1969.

Drusin, L. M., et al, "Electron Microscopy of *Treponema pallidum* Occurring in Human Primary Lesions." *Journal of Bacteriology,* 97:951, 1969.

Ducrey, A., "Recherches experimentales sur la Nature intime du principe contagieux du chancre mou." Annals Derm. Syph. (Par), 3 e Sér., 1:56, 1890.

Dunlop, E. M., et al, "Detection of Chlamydia (Bedsonia) in Certain Infections of Man, II. Clinical Study of Genital Tract, Eye, Rectum, and Other Sites of Recovery of Chlamydia." *Journal of Infectious Diseases,* 120:463, 1969.

Editorial, "Prophylaxis of Ophthalmia Neonatorum." *Jour-*

nal of the American Medical Association, 148:122, 1952.

Ellner, P. D., "The Occurrence of *Neisseria gonorrhoeae* in Routine Genital Cultures." *American Journal of Clinical Pathology,* 52:174, 1969.

Epstein, E., "Failure of Penicillin in Treatment of Acute Gonorrhea in American Troops in Korea." *Journal of the American Medical Association,* 169:1055, 1959.

Faigel, H. C., "Reported Patterns of Venereal Disease in Adolescents." *Clinical Pediatrics,* 8:620, 1969.

Fernando, W. L., "Erythromycin in Early Syphilis." *British Journal of Venereal Diseases,* 45:200.

Fisher, I., and Morton, R. S., "Epididymitis Due to *Trichomonas vaginalis.*" *British Journal of Venereal Diseases,* 45:252, 1969.

Fiumara, N. J., et al, "Venereal Diseases Today." *New England Journal of Medicine,* 260:863, 1959.

Fogel, B. J., et al, "Immunologic Response of the Fetus in Congenital Syphilis." *Journal of Florida Medical Association,* 56:777, 1969.

Forstrom, L., et al, "False Positive Reactions to the Reiter Protein Complement-Fixation (RPCF) Test." *British Journal of Venereal Diseases,* 45:126, 1969.

Friendly, D. S., "Gonococcal Conjunctivitis of the Newborn." *Clinical Proceedings of Children's Hospital, D. C.,* 25:1, 1969.

Gjessing, H. D., Odegaard, K., "Sensitivity of the Gonococcus to Antibiotics and Treatment of Gonorrhea 1,000 Cases)." *Acta Dermatovener (Stockh.),* 44:132, 1964.

Gjestland, T., "The Oslo Study of Untreated Syphilis: An Epidemiological Investigation of the Natural Course of Untreated Syphilitic Infections Based Upon a Restudy of The Boeck-Bruusgaard Material." *Acta Dermatovener (Stockh.)*, 35:Supplement 34, 1955

Greenwald, E., "Chancroidal Infection: Treatment and Diagnosis." *Journal of the American Medical Association,* 121:9, 1943.

Gundersen, T., et al, "Treatment of Gonorrhea by One Oral Dose of Ampicillin and Probenecid Combined." *British Journal of Venereal Diseases,* 45:235, 1969.

Halverson, C. A., et el, "*In-Vitro* Susceptibility of *N. gonorrhoeae* to Selected Antibiotics." *Military Medicine,* 139:1427, 1969.

Hanson, T., et al, "Gonorrheal Conjunctivitis, an Old Disease Returned." *Journal of the American Medical Association,* 195:1156, 1966.

Harris, A., et al, "Fluorescent Antibody Method of Detecting Gonorrhea in Asymptomatic Females." *Public Health Reports,* 76:93, 1961.

Harris, Ad., et al, "A Microflocculation Test for Syphilis Using Cardiolipin Antigen." Preliminary Report. *The Journal of Venereal Disease Information,* 27:169, 1946.

———. "The VDRL Slide Flocculation Test for Syphilis." *The Journal of Venereal Disease Information,* 29:72, 1948.

Hess, J., "Review of Current Methods for the Detection of Trichomonas in Clinical Material." *Journal of Clinical Pathology,* 22:269, 1969.

Heyman, A., et al, "Diagnosis of Chancroid; Relative Efficiency of Biopsies, Cultures, Smears, Autoinoculations and Skin Tests." *Journal of the American Medical Association,* 129:935, 1945.

Hirsch, H. A., and Finland, W., "Susceptibility of Gonococci to Antibiotics and Sulfadiazine." *American Journal of Medical Science,* 239:41, 1960.

Holmes, K. K., et al, "Studies of Venereal Disease: II. Observations on the Incidence, Etiology, and Treatment of the Post-Gonococcal Urethritis Syndrome." *Journal of the American Medical Association,* 202:461, 1967.

Hunter, E. F., "The Fluorescent Treponemal Antibody-Absorption (FTA-ABS) Test. Development, Use and Present Status." *Bulletin of World Health Organization,* 39:873, 1968.

"Increase in VD Triggers Alarm." *American Medical News,* Feb. (1971).

Jirovec, O., and Petu, M., "*Trichomonas vaginalis* and Trichomoniasis." *Advances in Parasitiology,* 6:117, 1968.

Johnson, D. W., et al, "An Evaluation of Gonorrhea Case Finding in the Chronically Infected Female." *American Journal of Epidemiology,* 90:438, 1969.

Josey, W. E., et al, "Viral and Virus-like Infections of the Female Genital Tract." *Clinical Obstetrics and Gynecology,* 12:161, 1969.

Juhlin, J., and Liden, S., "Influence of Contraceptive Gestogen Pills on Sexual Behavior and the Spread of Gonorrhoea." *British Journal of Venereal Diseases,* 45:321, 1969.

Kendell, H. W., et al, "Fever Therapy Technique in Syphilis and Gonococcic Infections." *Archives of Physical Medicine,* 50:603, 1969.

Kerber, R. E., et al, "Treatment of Chancroid. A Comparison of Tetracycline and Sulfisoxazole." *Archives of Dermatology,* 100:604, 1969.

Kercull, R. G., "Experiences With the Use of Sodium Ampicillin in Acute Gonococcal Infections in Vietnam." *Military Medicine,* 133:985, 1968.

Keyes, T. F., et al, "Single-dose Treatment of Gonorrhea

with Selected Antibiotic Agents." *Journal of the American Medical Association,* 210:857, 1969.

Kirsner, A. B., and Hess, E. V., "Gonococcal Arthritis." *Modern Treatment,* 6:1130, 1969.

Kjellander, J. O., "Penicillin Treatment of Gonorrheal Urethritis: Effects of Penicillin Susceptibility of Causative Organism and Concomitant Presence of Penicillinase-Producing Bacteria on Results." *New England Journal of Medicine,* 269:834, 1963.

Kradolfer, F., et al, "The Amoebicidal, Trichomonicidal, and Antibacterial Effects of Niridazole in Laboratory Animals." *Annals of New York Academy of Science,* 160:740, 1969.

Kraus, G. W., Yen, S. S. C., "Gonorrhea During Pregnancy." *Obstetrics and Gynecology,* 31:258, 1968.

Krook, G., and Juhlin, I., "Problems in Diagnosis, Treatment and Control of Gonorrheal Infections: IV. The Correlation Between the Dose of Penicillin, Concentrations in Blood, IC_{50}-Values of Gonococci and Results of Treatment." *Acta Dermatovener,* 45:242, 1965.

Kuhn, A. S. G., et al, "Experimental Pinta in the Chimpanzee." *Journal of the American Medical Association,* 206:829, 1968.

Kvale, P. A., et al, "Single Oral Dose Ampicillin-Probenecid Treatment of Gonorrhea in the Male." *Journal of the American Medical Association,* 215:1451, 1971.

Leigh, D. A., et al, "Sensitivity to Penicillin of *Neisseria gonorrhoeae.* Relationship to the Results of Treatment." *British Journal of Venereal Diseases,* 45:151, 1969.

Lenz, P. E., "Women, the Unwitting Carriers of Gonorrhea." *American Journal of Nursing,* 71:717, 1971.

Martin, J. E., Jr., et al, "Comparative Study of Gonococcal Susceptibility to Penicillin in Metropolitan Areas of the United States." Read before the Interscience Conference on Antimicrobial Agents and Chemotherapy, Washington, D. C., Oct. 27, 1969.

Martin, J. E., Jr., and Domescik, G., "Observations on the Culture Diagnosis of Gonorrhea in Women." *Journal of the American Medical Association,* 210:312, 1969.

Martin, J. E., Jr., and Lester, A., "Transgrow, A Medium for Transport and Growth of *Neisseria gonorrhoeae.*" *Public Health Reports.* In Press.

McDermott, W., "Microbial Persistence." *Yale Journal of Biological Medicine,* 30:257, 1958.

McFadzean, J. A., "Further Observations on Strain Sensitivity of *Trichomonas vaginalis* to Metronidazole." *British Journal of Venereal Diseases,* 45:161, 1969.

McGrew, B. E., "Quantitative Automated Reagin Test for Syphilis." *American Journal of Medical Technology,* 36:1, 1970.

Melnick, J. L., "Classification and Nomenclature of Animal Viruses, 1971." *Progr. med. Virol.,* 13:462, 1971.

Metzger, M., and Smogor, W., "Artificial Immunization of Rabbits Against Syphilis. Effect of Increasing Doses of Treponemes Given by the Intramuscular Route." *British Journal of Venereal Diseases,* 45:308, 1969.

Metzger, M., et al, "Immunologic Properties of the Protein Component of Treponema pallidum." *British Journal of Venereal Diseases.* 45:299, 1969.

Moore, M. B., "The Epidemiology of Syphilis." *Journal of the American Medical Association,* 186:71, 1963.

Nahmias, A. J., et al, "Genital Infection with Type 2

Herpesvirus hominis. A Commonly Occurring Venereal Disease." *British Journal of Venereal Diseases,* 45:294, 1969.

———. "Newborn Infection with Herpesvirus hominis Types 1 and 2." *Journal of Pediatrics,* 75:1194, 1969.

Nelson, M., "Comparative Study of Two Therapies for Gonorrhea." *Public Health Reports,* 84:980, 1969.

Nemec, F., "The Treatment of Gonorrhea With a Single High-Dosed Penicillin Injection (So-called "One-Shot" Treatment)." *Z. Haut Geschlechtskr,* 44:507, 1969.

O'Brien, J. T., "The Laboratory Diagnosis of Gonorrhoea in the Female." *New Zealand Medical Journal,* 69:204, 1969.

Olsen, G. G. A., and Lomholt, G., "Gonorrhoea Treatment by a Combination of Probenecid and Sodium Penicillin." *British Journal of Venereal Diseases,* 45:144, 1969.

Pariser, H., and Marino, A., "Gonorrhea—Frequently Unrecognized Reservoirs." *Southern Medical Journal,* 63:198, 1970.

"Patterns of Venereal Disease Morbidity in Recent Years." *Statistics Bulletin of the Metropolitan Life Insurance Co.,* 50:5, 1969.

Phillips, I., et al, "In-vitro Activity of Twelve Antibacterial Agents Against *Neisseria gonorrheae.*" *Lancet,* 1:263, 1970.

Prewitt, T. A., "Syphilitic Aortic Insufficiency. Its Increased Incidence in the Elderly." *Journal of the American Medical Association,* 211:637, 1970.

Rawlins, D. C., "Drug-taking by Patients With Venereal Disease." *British Journal of Venereal Diseases,* 45:238, 1969.

Rawls, W. E., et al, "Herpes Type 2: Association With Carcinoma of the Cervix." *Science*, 161:1255, 1968.

Rees, E., and Annels, E. H., "Gonococcal Salpingitis." *British Journal of Venereal Diseases*, 45:205, 1969.

Reyn, A., "Recent Developments in the Laboratory Diagnosis of Gonococcal Infections." *Bulletin of World Health Organization*, 40:245, 1969.

Robinson, R. C. V., "Congenital Syphilis." *Archives Dermatology*, 99:599, 1969.

Ronald, J. E., et al, "Susceptibility of *Neisseria gonorrhoeae* to Penicillin and Tetracycline." *Antimicrobial Agents Chemotherapy*, 8:431, 1968.

Satulsky, E. M., "Management of Chancroid in a Tropical Theater; Report of 1555 Cases." *Journal of the American Medical Association*, 127:259, 1945.

Schachter, D. E., et al, "Lymphogranuloma venereum. Comparison of the Frei Test, Complement Fixation Test, and Isolation of the Agent." *Journal of Infectious Diseases*, 120:372, 1969.

Schmale, J. D., "Observations on Culture Diagnosis of Gonorrhea in Women." *Journal of the American Medical Association*, 210:312, 1969.

Schmale, J. D., et al, "Isolation of an Antigen of *Neisseria gonorrhoeae* Involved in the Human Immune Response to Gonococcal Infection." *Journal of Bacteriology*, 99:469, 1969.

Schofield, C. B., "Medicosocial Background to Gonococcal Ophthalmia Neonatorum." *Lancet*, 2:1182, 1969.

Schroetter, A. L., and Pazin, G. J., "Gonorrhea-Diagnosis and Treatment." *Annals of Internal Medicine*, 72:555, 1970.

Scott, J., and Stone, A. H., "Some Observations on the Diagnosis of Rectal Gonorrhea in Both Sexes Using

Selective Culture Medium." *British Journal of Venereal Diseases,* 42:103, 1966.

Scotti, A., Logan, L., and Caldwell, J. G., "Fluorescent Antibody Test for Neonatal Congenital Syphilis: A Progress Report." *Journal of Pediatrics,* 75:1129, 1969.

Shapiro, L. H., "Gonorrhea in Females." Philadelphia, Venereal Disease Control Section, Public Health Department. (No date.)

Smith, J. A., "Ophthalmia Neonatorum in Glasgow." *Scottish Medical Journal,* 14:272, 1969.

Smith, L. J., "The Current Status of Ocular Syphilis." *Survey of Ophthalmology,* 14:176, 1969.

Spaeth, G. M., "Treatment of Penicillin Resistant Gonorrheal Conjunctivitis with Ampicillin." *American Journal of Ophthalmology,* 66:427, 1968.

Stevens, R. W., and Stroekel, E., "The Automated Reagin Test: Results Compared with VDRL and FTA-ABS." *American Journal of Clinical Pathology,* 53:32, 1970.

Svihus, R. H., "Gonorrhea-like Syndrome Caused by Penicillin-Resistant Mimeae." *Journal of the American Medical Association,* 177:121, 1961.

Thatcher, R. W., and Pettit, T. H., "Gonorrheal Conjunctivitis." *Journal of the American Medical Association,* 215:1494, 1971.

Thatcher, R. W., et al, "Asymptomatic Gonorrhea." *Journal of the American Medical Association,* 210:315, 1969.

———. "Gonorrheal Urethritis in Males Treated with Single Oral Dose of Minocycline." *Public Health Reports,* 85:158, 1970.

Thayer, J. D., "Comparative Antibiotic Susceptibility of *N. Gonorrhoeae* from 1955 to 1964." *Antimicrobial Agents and Chemotherapy,* 1964:433, 1965.

Thayer, J. D., and Axnick, N. W., "Susceptibility of Gonococci to Ten Penicillins." *Antimicrobial Agents and Chemotherapy,* 1963:427, 1964.

Thayer, J. D., and Kellogg, D. S., Jr., "Virulence of Gonococci." *Annual Review of Medicine,* 20:323, 1969.

Thew, M. A., "Ampicillin in the Treatment of Granuloma Inguinale." *Journal of the American Medical Association,* 210:866, 1969.

"Today's VD Control Problem: A Joint Statement by the American Public Health Association, American Social Health Association and American Venereal Disease Association." New York, American Social Health Association, 1970.

"Today's VD Control Problem—1971. New York, American Social Health Association, 1971.

Turner, T. B., "Infectivity Tests in Syphilis." *British Journal of Venereal Diseases,* 45:183, 1969.

Turner, T. B., and Hollander, D. H., "Biology of the Treponematoses." Geneva: Monopaper Series No. 35, World Health Organization.

Vandermeer, D. C., "Meet the VD Epidemiologist." *American Journal of Nursing,* 71:722, 1971.

Wallace, A. L., "Trends and Uses of Various Tests in Syphilis Serology Today." *Technical Bulletin of the Registry of Medical Technologists,* 35:712, 1965.

Willcox, R. R., "Treatment of Gonorrhoea with Double Doses of Demethylchlortetracycline." *Acta Dermatovener,* 49:103, 1969.

Wilmer, H. A., "Corky the Killer (A Story of Syphilis)." New York: American Social Hygiene Association, 1950.

Index

Page numbers in *italics* indicate illustrations.